BETH SHAW'S YOGAFIT®

Second Edition

Beth Shaw

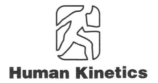

Human Kinetics

Library of Congress Cataloging-in-Publication Data

Shaw, Beth.
  [YogaFit]
  Beth Shaw's Yogafit® / Beth Shaw. -- 2nd ed.
    p. cm.
  Includes index.
  ISBN-13: 978-0-7360-7536-7 (soft cover)
  ISBN-10: 0-7360-7536-4 (soft cover)
 1. Physical fitness. 2. Hatha yoga. I. Title.
  RA781.7.S446 2009
  613.7'046--dc22

                                2008037999

ISBN-10: 0-7360-7536-4
ISBN-13: 978-0-7360-7536-7

This publication is written and published to provide accurate and authoritative information relevant to the subject matter presented. It is published and sold with the understanding that the author and publisher are not engaged in rendering legal, medical, or other professional services by reason of their authorship or publication of this work. If medical or other expert assistance is required, the services of a competent professional person should be sought.

The Web addresses cited in this text were current as of August 2008, unless otherwise noted.

Acquisitions Editor: Tom Heine; **Project Consultant:** Katie Pearson; **Developmental Editor:** Laura Floch; **Assistant Editors:** Laura Podeschi and Elizabeth Watson; **Copyeditor:** John Wentworth; **Proofreader:** Kathy Bennett; **Graphic Designer:** Joe Buck; **Graphic Artist:** Kim McFarland; **Cover Designer:** Keith Blomberg; **Photographer (cover and interior):** Victoria Davis; **Visual Production Assistant:** Joyce Brumfield; **Photo Production Manager:** Jason Allen; **Art Manager:** Kelly Hendren; **Associate Art Manager:** Alan L. Wilborn; **Illustrator:** Bullseye Studio; **Printer:** United Graphics

We thank Victoria Davis Studios in Santa Monica, California, for assistance in providing the location for the photo shoot for this book.

Human Kinetics books are available at special discounts for bulk purchase. Special editions or book excerpts can also be created to specification. For details, contact the Special Sales Manager at Human Kinetics.

Printed in the United States of America   10   9   8   7   6   5   4   3

The paper in this book is certified under a sustainable forestry program.

Human Kinetics
Web site: www.HumanKinetics.com

United States: Human Kinetics, P.O. Box 5076, Champaign, IL 61825-5076
800-747-4457
email: humank@hkusa.com

Canada: Human Kinetics, 475 Devonshire Road Unit 100, Windsor, ON N8Y 2L5
800-465-7301 (in Canada only)
email: info@hkcanada.com

Europe: Human Kinetics, 107 Bradford Road, Stanningley, Leeds LS28 6 AT, United Kingdom
+44 (0) 113 255 5665
email: hk@hkeurope.com

Australia: Human Kinetics, 57A Price Avenue, Lower Mitcham, South Australia 5062
08 8372 0999
e-mail: info@hkaustralia.com

New Zealand: Human Kinetics, Division of Sports Distributors NZ Ltd., P.O. Box 300 226 Albany,
North Shore City, Auckland
0064 9 448 1207
e-mail: info@humankinetics.co.nz

For Renee Taylor, YogaFit staff and trainers,
and the vast community of friends and enthusiasts

CONTENTS

Part III Putting It All Together 199

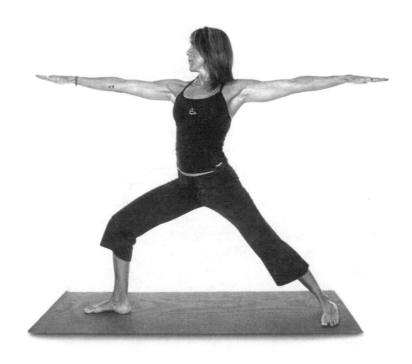

FOREWORDS

At the Applied Neuroscience Institute we are dedicated to taking sophisticated theories and research and simplifying and integrating them into concrete methods that lead to helping people "feel good." Our work is at the crossroads of neuroscience, positive psychology, and quantum physics so we're always interested in finding people who have integrated approaches that affect people on a number of levels. Beth Shaw and YogaFit understand something about this integration of methods that is very unusual. But, as it is said, the proof is in the pudding.

I had the opportunity to address the corporate board of YogaFit and then to present my own work called *The Emotional Gym* to their trainers. More than any other group I have worked with, they *get it*. As soon as I started to talk about integrating emotion and movement and then feeling good, they were with me in a way that let me know that YogaFit is for real—not just an exercise program but a holistic model of personal growth that aims at much more than a fit body. YogaFit, in its levels of experience, is about feeling good on levels of human experience that last and create personal flourishing over time. In other words, you flourish and get lasting results over the long haul.

Beth Shaw is doing something that is rare. Too often we think that Eastern practices or esoteric practices of personal growth translate immediately or effectively into Western culture. They do not, and because they don't, they don't last except with a group of niche followers or devotees. What Beth has done is build a model that is for everybody, that is applicable, that works, and that lasts over time. Beth has developed a program for living a fuller life that is solid and definitive but able to be experienced in a very individual way. You are not molded to a program; YogaFit is molded and formed for you.

Let's face it—many exercise programs today are boring and shallow. Others advertise that they integrate body and mind, but such integration doesn't happen without a plan. For most of these programs it's a hope, not a reality. You put in your time, feel a little high from the exercise, and check the mirror too often to see what difference it has made. YogaFit is about the change from the inside to the outside. This is why when I encountered the YogaFit trainers I met vitally alive people—alive to themselves and alive to life. They were about helping people living optimal lives, and they were an example of that vitality. They did not represent an elitist program for a healthy few, but a grass-roots, down-to-earth, "we care about you" program that makes everyone feel that they belong and that they can succeed. As Beth Shaw says, "If you can breathe, you can do yoga."

This is a program about integrating levels of experience toward a simple goal: to be fit and to *feel good*. Beth Shaw realizes an important thing in exercise, that being fit doesn't necessarily mean feeling good. She understands that fitness involves many levels of human experience. She has developed a program of integrated methodologies that makes yoga accessible to everyone. This integration of diverse methodologies with a sense of fitness is at the heart of YogaFit and makes it a distinct stand-alone program quite apart from the fitness circus the average person doesn't choose because he or she doesn't know what to trust. You can trust this one, and you can believe in YogaFit because fitness is understood here in a unique combination of body, mind, and spirit that fits the culture of the Western world and suits a journey not just to disciplines but to the heart of the matter of fitness. It's a journey toward feeling good.

Dr. William Kent Larkin
Director
Applied Neuroscience Institute
Author, *Growing the Positive Mind*

At first glance, it might seem that yoga, with its nearly 20 million practitioners in the United States, hasn't a lot in common with organized animal protection. But that's a mistaken assumption. The two movements are ascendant and share a host of intersections, especially today, in an era marked by extraordinary threats to personal and planetary health.

It's not a surprise to find the yoga world populated with people like Beth Shaw, who has a wonderful passion for animals, who acts as an ambassador for animals and their interests, and who gets personally involved in the prevention of cruelty.

Yoga brings tremendous personal health benefits, as those who practice it work to improve and maintain their bodies and their minds, and to achieve a spiritual centeredness. However, the philosophy and practice of yoga also involves a concept of social health. Its practitioners know that personal health and personal change involve greater self-awareness, yet they also live with an understanding that such awareness will lead to a broader social change for the good.

Animal protection also proceeds from a focus on the individual to a broader focus on the social. At its most elemental level, the work of The Humane Society of the United States (HSUS) is about protecting individual beings—nonhuman animals—and about creating a broader social awareness that ensures their well-being and safety. Whether it's changing our diets to help animals and to mitigate the impact of livestock agriculture on climate change, or adopting animals from a shelter rather than purchasing them from a pet store or puppy mill, or instructing young children in the lessons of kindness and mindfulness of others, we are all playing a part in securing a greater measure of social health, as well as doing ourselves some good.

In reading this important book, it occurred to me that the yamas and niyamas of yoga are as good a set of guidelines for living as you'll find, and they embody the richness of yoga as a philosophy and practice. What's more, they're highly consistent with a concern for animals. One of the five yamas, Ahimsa, dynamic harmlessness, has long been a cornerstone of humane philosophy, and it's a term as familiar to animal protectionists as to yoga enthusiasts.

In the realm of animal protection, the path of selfless service and giving is a long and winding road. The needs are great, the challenges are daunting, and the frustrations can be high. Both I and my colleagues at the HSUS, the nation's largest animal protection organization, feel these pressures so deeply each and every day.

Whenever I feel overwhelmed, I have only to remind myself that there are millions of people out there trying to do their part, and it especially helps me to know that there are people like Beth, whose vitality, openness, and healthy attitudes about life and its challenges are inspiring.

As I've learned more about Beth's devotion to the cause of animals, I've wondered about the source of her boundless energy, her optimism, and her can-do spirit. Now I know that it comes from yoga and the principles she shares in this book. By her own account, yoga has enhanced her life in the fullest way. I hope it does the same for you.

Wayne Pacelle
President & CEO
Humane Society of the United States

PREFACE

One of the primary attractions for Westerners to YogaFit is that you don't have to change your life to receive the rewards—YogaFit is compatible with your lifestyle today. Although traditional yoga has much to offer, it isn't necessary to speak Sanskrit (the original language of key yoga texts), chant, or even become vegetarian to enjoy the multidimensional benefits of this ancient practice. Nor do you have to be flexible or familiar with any aspect of yoga to begin. In fact, inflexibility is one of the primary reasons this program is so effective, particularly for active individuals and athletes who need to round out their strength-training routines. Whether you're just beginning to discover the benefits of exercise, or you've been working out for years, YogaFit will enrich your exercise program and your ability to enjoy life. Most people discover that the more they study and practice YogaFit, the more they want to make healthier choices and alter their lifestyle to support feeling and living better.

As with any lifestyle change, slow and steady wins the race. As you read, take time to absorb what captures your attention. Stop and savor, just as you would during a YogaFit pose (as you will learn); don't push through and rush the process just to get to the last chapter. Know that not only can you go back and reread sections that interested you or escaped you on the first reading, but that you should revisit the information regularly, until it becomes part of you. Embrace the idea that once the process of growth and change has begun, it will see itself through to the end. Be patient with yourself and the process.

In this book you will find many of the components of traditional yoga presented in a way that allows you to explore and adopt what you like, when you like. Part I, *Preparing to Be YogaFit*, focuses on the program's philosophy, from how the actual workouts are structured, to breathing practices, to traditional guidelines that teach healthier ways of interacting both with ourselves and the world we live in. It might be tempting to gloss over this information and skip right to the poses, but resist doing so. These chapters come first because to be effective yoga must be regarded through a different lens than traditional exercise. There is no competition. Your breath sets the pace. Honoring your body's need for rest is just as important as knowing when to push—maybe more so. By reading and absorbing part I, you will enhance your understanding of the poses and how to practice them for maximum enjoyment and benefit.

Part II, *Purposeful Poses*, makes up the majority of the book. The poses are classified according to general position: standing, balancing, forward bending, backward bending, and so on. These chapters are meant to be read in their entirety before you attempt a YogaFit session because a well-rounded workout draws poses from each of these chapters.

Part III, *Putting It All Together*, takes the confusion out of how to select and combine poses by offering several class formats for beginning, intermediate, and experienced practitioners. We've also included poses that complement specific sports and activities. This allows you to feel confident starting your YogaFit journey, while giving you the freedom to eventually create your own workouts based on your personal needs and interests.

As Beth's story in the Introduction will indicate, this book is quite literally for everybody and every *body,* with the exception of those with special or chronic conditions. As with any exercise program, before beginning your YogaFit practice, please check with your doctor to ensure that this program is safe for you. What separates YogaFit from other forms of exercise is that YogaFit speaks directly and without pretentiousness to everyone, helping you and your body reach their potential.

INTRODUCTION

Fitness has always held high appeal for me. To this day I enjoy few things more than moving my body in some way, be it dancing, walking my dogs, working out, or doing yoga. Since I was very young, I swam and moved around a lot. Being an only child, I was never much into team sports, preferring solitary activities like running, swimming, and biking. I feel so blessed that although I grew up in New York City, I was able to develop a love for all things physical. I started working out at health clubs when I was 15.

Through college I worked out with friends, doing aerobics (which I was never good at) and playing tennis (marginal). I belonged to a gym where I made friends with a bodybuilder named Gary. One day at the gym I had a psychic flash while stretching. The sky seemed to part with a white light, and the message came to me that I would one day be successful in the fitness industry.

After college, I moved from New York to California, where I unwittingly started a sedentary advertising sales job. I promptly gained 40 pounds. Soon after, I decided I better get things together, so I joined Gold's Gym and began going every morning at 5 o'clock. Gradually, things in my life took a turn. I swapped bean and cheese burritos for carrot sticks and hard-boiled eggs. I took control of my credit card debt and student loans. I found myself growing stronger emotionally and mentally. Exercise was literally turning my life around.

When I moved to L.A., yoga was one of those seemingly "California" things I always wanted to try, like getting a waterbed and a cell phone. My first yoga teacher was Renee Taylor. After being diagnosed with cancer in the 1960s Renee had gone to live in Rishikesh, the birthplace of yoga at the basin of the Ganges River in the Himalayas. She learned the many aspects of yoga, adopted a vegetarian diet . . . and was healed. She came home and started teaching yoga, writing books, and making tapes. I have had the opportunity to visit Rishikesh in recent years and am constantly amazed by the incredible energy of the region and the effect that simply "being there" has on me.

Renee was well into her 90s when I met her. She would just sit on her desk in her carpeted studio and instruct. We did yoga on beach towels back then. I was a runner at the time, and she used to tell me, "Don't run, just do yoga." But I was initially awkward in most of my attempts. Slowly, my practice improved, and over time I mastered some poses. Visiting yoga ashrams and retreats gave me a glimpse into the more esoteric aspects of the practice. I made a whole group of yoga friends; we would attend classes and take trips together. I had found a group of like-minded people, and I look back on those days as some of my most profound. Yoga came first. I was disciplined and focused on my practice. My yoga practice led me to become a spiritual seeker. Personal growth workshops, astrology, movement expression—you name it, I did it. I looked under every rock for an answer, a spiritual experience, and a connection.

In 1993 I took my first of many teacher trainings. I was soon teaching several classes a week at a variety of health clubs. It felt only right that in my teaching I would blend my love and knowledge of fitness with my yoga teachings. Students loved it! We played fun music, incorporated fitness moves, and everyone felt good. Not long after, I started producing a local cable TV yoga show called YogaFit. (The name came to me on a bike ride.)

Around that time my second yoga teacher left our health club to open her own studio. The manager of the club approached me to turn the club's golf room into a yoga studio. In 1994 we opened what I believe was the first yoga studio within a health club in the United States. By that time I was selling my YogaFit logo wear in my classes and had really gotten the name out in the South Bay of Los Angeles. Yoga magazines were writing up my clothing and TV show, and I had produced an audiotape for an audio book company. Seeing the brand's potential, one of my yoga students, Po Chang, took a chance, invested seed money into YogaFit, and helped me incorporate. The term Angel Investor is indeed an accurate one; I could not have done any of this without his vision and support.

I opened my first YogaFit studio in early 1998. Community service was just as important to us then as it is now; we held breast cancer fundraisers, pet adoptions, and children's classes. I've always felt that no matter how big or small your business is, it is important to give back. How rich or poor you feel is all relative, and we all have the power to make a positive difference on this planet in some way. To negate or ignore this natural calling and duty is to deny the essence and beauty of being a human (humane) being.

Yoga has changed my life in every possible way you can imagine, and in many ways that no one can. I am grateful to the practice daily—grateful for the opportunity to move, to breathe, to feel; grateful to be able to assist others in transformation, evolution, and awakening; grateful to be able to witness positive change in myself and others around me; grateful for the beautiful spirits that work for YogaFit and their desire to move themselves and others toward the light; grateful to have this energetic wave called YogaFit that has changed millions of lives; grateful for the opportunity to keep growing within my own yoga practice; grateful for the calling (dharma) to help animals; and grateful that YogaFit provides me the opportunity to support the animal movement in so many ways.

In his book *Growing the Positive Mind*, Dr. William K. Larkin says that the body chemistry associated with gratitude is the most optimally healthy state of mind. Research shows that a positive state of mind affects us at a cellular level. When practicing yoga, be grateful for what you can do, and the rest will come in time—when it's right, and when you are ready. The physical body is perhaps the most tangible testing ground we have. As in YogaFit's education ladder, everything starts with the physical—from there we grow and transcend.

May we always approach our physical practice with this deep appreciation— to be in these bodies, to move, to breathe, to feel, to sweat—what a gift.

Namasté—
Beth

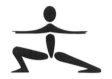

Part I

Preparing to Be YogaFit

1

YogaFit Essentials

Welcome to your yoga journey. One of the beautiful things about yoga is that you can do it just about anywhere and any time. You can be indoors or outdoors; you can take it with you when you travel or do it in the office or on a plane, boat, or train. In a moment we'll discuss ways to incorporate YogaFit into your life, but first let's look at why this program has become a way of life for so many people.

THE BENEFITS OF YOGAFIT

A regular YogaFit workout, as you'll see in chapter 10, gives you all the benefits of a traditional yoga practice and more. Best results are achieved by practicing three to five times a week for 30 to 60 minutes per workout. The more you practice YogaFit, the more benefits you receive, though most people experience a positive difference after just one workout. The benefits of YogaFit are many, including

- increased flexibility,
- stronger muscles,
- better body tone,
- a naturally defined physique,
- a relaxed and clear mind,
- reduced stress,
- increased body awareness,
- natural weight loss,
- improved posture,

- a strengthened immune system, and
- decreased physical effects of aging for the brain and body.

Along with the benefits of a traditional yoga practice, a regular YogaFit workout also helps you succeed in your athletic endeavors by reducing the risk of injury through a greater mind–body connection; creating a more effective metabolic exchange during physical activity via better breathing patterns; offsetting the unevenness of other exercise programs by offering a complete and balanced mind–body workout for all muscle groups; and increasing endurance, willpower, and discipline by working both your body and your mind (see chapter 10 for details on using YogaFit to cross train with your favorite sports).

PREPARING FOR YOUR YOGAFIT WORKOUT

Before you begin, let's look at ways to create an optimal atmosphere for your yoga experience.

> Your body is different every day, so be aware of your body's needs and requirements before, during, and after your YogaFit session. Over time you'll learn what's best for your body at any given moment. Until then relax and try to listen to your body at all times.

Know your limits. It's probably best to read this entire book before you jump into your YogaFit program, but for success and safety before your first workout be sure to read at least all of part I, all of chapter 10 (which presents balanced workout formats), and the descriptions of any poses in part II that you want to try. Before starting this program or any other new workout, be sure to check with your physician, especially if you have injuries, special conditions, or chronic illnesses, or if you are pregnant, over 65, or not currently participating in a regular exercise program. Also see "Special Considerations for YogaFit" at the end of this chapter for ideas on how to modify your workout in accordance with your condition.

Take your time. Reread sections of this book until you absorb all that YogaFit has to offer. Don't feel rushed. You'll benefit most by going slowly through your first session at your own pace. Stop for breaks when you need them.

Allow time for meals and snacks to digest. Before beginning your yoga session allow at least 90 minutes after a meal so that your body has time to digest. If you feel you need a snack during that 90 minutes, choose fruit, tea, or an energy drink. Just make sure you consume these at least 30 minutes before you begin.

Stop all other activity at least 15 minutes before each practice.
Use the time before your session to calm, collect, and center yourself. This is a good time to prepare the room. Turn off (or tone down) harsh lighting. Light candles and play music to create an atmosphere that helps you focus. You'll want to leave your everyday thoughts behind, as discussed later in this chapter.

Position in an open space away from mirrors.
Roll out your mat with enough space to allow room for your arms and legs to move freely. Avoid being too close to walls, doors, or furniture. Don't face mirrors because they draw your focus away from how your body feels (you'll focus on how you look instead). Relax your face into a natural smile. Consciously release any holding patterns in your face, neck, and shoulders. Make adjustments that seem right to you. You want your YogaFit session to be an enjoyable experience that you want to return to.

Maintain a positive mental attitude.
For success with your YogaFit session, begin with an open mind. The practice of yoga is a fluid one, a lifelong journey of change and transformation. Your practice might change from one day to the next, but maintain faith in the process. As with any exercise program, you'll see and feel results over time. A positive attitude is an important part of your practice because your thoughts directly influence your body chemistry and immune system. What you think determines whether you are working for your body or against it.

Know your range of motion and flexibility.
We all want to be like bamboo, strong but flexible, but each body is different in type, flexibility, and fitness level. Therefore, two people looking alike in the same pose is not likely. A "perfect fit" varies from person to person. This variety is an aspect of yoga that keeps things interesting—you're always trying to learn what works best for your own body.

> No two bodies respond to the same stretch in exactly the same way. *Remember that you want to make the pose fit your body, not your body fit the pose.* Never force, push or shove yourself into a pose. Instead use breathing techniques (chapter 3) to enhance your practice.

Note that if you have an unusually limited range of motion you should focus on proper alignment and breathing rather than on achieving maximum flexibility. Use the modifications in part II to work muscle groups without strain or risk of injury.

YogaFit's Seven Principles of Alignment

In YogaFit we express yoga postures in terms of what we call the Seven Principles of Alignment (SPA). These principles help create the optimal biomechanical positioning for your body during movement and while you're holding your YogaFit poses. SPA increases safety while providing functional mechanical principles that you can apply in your daily life. Let's look at a brief explanation for each of the seven principles.

1. *Establish Base and Dynamic Tension*

   For maximum stability, mobility, and extension, build your poses from the ground up by establishing a firm foundation. If your hands are on the mat, spread your fingers wide. If your feet are on the mat, distribute your weight evenly across your feet and press down to form a strong base. Next, stack your joints. For example, if you're on all fours, align your shoulders over your wrists and your hips over your knees. This allows you to build strength in alignment and protect your joints from injury. Finally, contract your muscles and extend outward through your limbs and the crown of your head. This creates dynamic tension, which increases your energy and effectiveness in every pose. For example, in Warrior II (p. 78) you reach out in opposite directions through your fingers while reaching up through the crown of your head and sinking into the lunge.

2. *Create Core Stability*

   The muscles of your midsection (abdominals, lower back, glutes, hip flexors) make up your core. Engage these muscles before moving into and while holding poses to create strength, stability, and mobility. When you work from a stable core you can move with confidence into your poses—and hold them with greater ease.

3. *Align the Spine*

   The spine is supported through core stabilization. When moving into twists, side bends, forward bends, or backward bends, always start by engaging your core and finding your neutral (straight) spine. This strengthens your muscles in alignment and helps prevent injury. Remember that the head and neck are part of the spine and always follow the movement of the spine. Aligning the spine builds strength in alignment and prevents increasing tension in your neck and shoulders.

4. *Soften and Align the Knees*

   In any standing pose in which one or both legs is straight, keep a soft bend in the knee (or knees) to avoid locking out the joint. In YogaFit, we call this a "microbend." The slight bend helps stabilize and protect the joint by strengthening surrounding muscles and corrects any muscular imbalances in the legs. Refer to poses such as Warrior I (p.

76), Kneeling or Crescent Lunge (p. 166), and Chair (p. 88), in which you stack your knees above your ankles and point them directly over your toes. In general, the knees, when bent, remain in the same line as the hips.

5. *Relax Shoulders Back and Down*

   When stressed, fatigued, or tense, your shoulders tend to rise up toward your ears, which increases tension in your upper body and decreases core stability. So, in any pose, even those with arms overhead such as in Warrior I (p. 76), or with hands on the mat as in Downward-Facing Dog (p. 108), slide your shoulder blades toward your hip pockets and draw the tips toward your spine to open your chest.

6. *Hinge at the Hips*

   When moving into and out of forward bends, bend your knees and hinge at your hips, using the natural pulley system of your hip joints. This will allow you to maintain a neutral spine and prevent injuries to your lower back. Also use this movement in daily activities such as when lifting objects or bending over.

7. *Shorten the Lever*

   When hip hinging, flexing, or extending your spine, keep your arms out to your sides or alongside your body to reduce the load placed on the muscles of your lower back. Bend your elbows instead of using straight arms. Any position can be used as long as your arms are not lifted next to the ears with elbows fully extended. For example, when moving from Standing Forward Fold (p. 106) back to Mountain (p. 66), "circle sweep" your arms around and up instead of reaching directly forward. Or, in Locust (p. 136), keep your arms back alongside your body instead of in front of you.

WHAT YOU NEED TO BEGIN YOGAFIT

Let's discuss what you need to begin your program. For more information on many of the products discussed in this section, refer to appendix B (p. 271).

Clothing

Wear comfortable and snug but nonbinding clothing. You'll be sweating and stretching when you practice, and your skin tends to absorb what's next to it, so consider organic bamboo or organic cotton clothing. Shirts that are too loose will ride up during certain poses, so women often prefer tank tops with built-in sports bras, tights, flex pants, or capris. Men wear shorts, tank tops, or long-sleeve T-shirts. Layering is a good idea because you'll warm up and cool down. And don't forget: no shoes, no socks. YogaFit is best done barefoot.

A Yoga Mat

There are many yoga mats on the market with slick surfaces that quickly deteriorate. To ensure you get a quality mat with staying power, buy from a vendor that specializes in yoga accessories. Because your body will often be in direct contact with your mat, consider an eco-friendly or organic mat. These mats are also better for the environment.

You can decide for yourself if you want a thin mat or a thick mat. Some prefer thin mats because they're almost like practicing directly on the floor surface, allowing for maximum stability. But thick mats provide extra cushioning and often are best for people with knee discomfort on hard floors.

A Hard Surface

For your YogaFit session, place your mat on a wooden floor or another hard, flat, and smooth surface. You want a firm foundation that offers balance and provides optimal alignment for your joints.

Props

Props include blocks, straps, chairs, rolled-up yoga mats or blankets, and even walls. Without props, many people can't get the full benefits of the YogaFit poses. Props aren't necessarily intended to make poses easier; rather, they allow you to find a position that you can hold longer without overstretching or straining so you can focus on increasing strength and flexibility. Props can also help you overcome hesitancy and find balance, thereby boosting your confidence and promoting a feeling of success—without which you might not return to your mat.

The props listed here can make the YogaFit poses safe and effective for everyone, no matter your body type (see appendix B for details on where to purchase these items).

- *Blocks.* Blocks are lightweight foam bricks or wooden blocks used in poses in which tightness or unsteadiness prevents you from reaching the floor without overstretching or coming out of alignment. In these poses, you place one or both hands on a block.
- *Straps.* Yoga straps are useful for people with limited flexibility or injury concerns. Straps allow you to practice a pose that might otherwise be impossible or difficult, allowing you to realize the benefits of the pose with comfort. We've indicated in the pose chapters when a strap might be helpful to modify a pose. If you don't own a strap, use a bathrobe belt or a necktie.
- *Chair.* A chair is useful for added height for forward movements, for balance, and for simple inversions.
- *Mats or blankets.* Place a mat or blanket under your head, knees, or lower back for support in positions in which you lie on your back. You can also

sit on a rolled-up mat or folded blanket to lift your hips in seated forward folds to maintain a straight spine.

- *Walls.* Use a wall for support during standing balance and simple inversions.
- *Knee pads.* If you have sensitive knees, place a folded towel under your kneecaps, or cut an old yoga mat into strips to place over your mat for extra padding during kneeling poses.

Other Items

Yoga is a personal experience. You want to create an environment for your practice that invites you back. You can do this in many ways. We offer some suggestions, but also have fun experimenting with what motivates or inspires you to make your workout feel as if you're "coming home."

Music

Although some people opt not to play music so they can focus only on the sound of their breathing, a good CD that matches the tone of your practice is often helpful for inspiration and motivation.

YogaFit provides many options for music so that you can find a style that suits you and your workout, from ambient music without lyrics (my personal favorite because it energizes without distracting) to a variety of styles and mixes with vocals. There are many "active" and zen series CDs formatted to match the three mountains of a YogaFit workout (see chapter 4). These begin with slower music, progress to more upbeat music in the middle, then wind down in tempo for deep stretches and Final Relaxation. Using these CDs, you need not switch out your music in the middle of your practice.

Aromatherapy

Natural essential oils in a diffuser create a pleasing setting and a scent awareness during your YogaFit session. If you haven't used essential oils, we recommend sticking to the basics to help you get started. You can find these oils at any natural food store.

- Lavender is widely known for its soothing and relaxing effect on the mind—perfect for winding down after a hard day.
- Eucalyptus has a cooling and stimulating effect on the mind and body. Use this oil when you need an energy boost for your practice.
- Ylang ylang has a beautiful floral scent and is known to relax your mind, lift your spirits, and perhaps lower blood pressure caused by stress. Use this oil when practicing restorative yoga.
- Sandalwood has been used for over 4,000 years in Hindu ceremonies and is still used today for medicinal purposes and to calm nerves and decrease anxiety.

• Patchouli, a beautiful scent with hints of orange and amber, reduces anxiety and relaxes your mind.

Candles

Candles give an ambient glow and can provide a focal point that's beneficial for standing balance poses. Use soy candles that burn without toxic fumes (see appendix B).

SPECIAL CONSIDERATIONS FOR YOGAFIT

Take care to modify your YogaFit sessions with special conditions such as pregnancy, injury, or other medical conditions. Note that inverted poses and backbends are for advanced students after a vigorous warm-up only.

Injuries or Medical Conditions

Here is a list of common injuries and medical conditions for which you will likely need to modify your YogaFit workout:

• *Sciatica.* Bend your knees in forward folds. Avoid intense hamstring stretches.

• *Hypertension (high blood pressure).* Avoid holding your breath; avoid inverted postures.

• *Glaucoma or other eye problems.* Avoid holding your breath; avoid inverted postures.

• *Sinus infections, ear infections, congestion.* Avoid holding your breath; avoid inverted postures.

• *Back or neck injuries.* Avoid inverted postures.

• *Knee problems.* Avoid quad stretches; do the Upside Down Pigeon with extra care. Use knee pads or place extra padding under the knees for floor work.

• *Wrist problems.* Make "fists" for wrists (palms facing each other) in any pose in which shoulders are stacked directly above the wrists, such as the Incline Plank, Cat/Cow, Spinal Balance, or Tabletop.

• *Shoulder injuries.* Avoid raising your arms for extended periods, such as in Warrior II or Chair. Also avoid poses that place a heavy load on your shoulders, such as the Crocodile and Plank poses, or drop your knees when performing these poses. Also keep hands directly under pectorals in Crocodile or Plank poses to support your shoulders.

Pregnancy

Although yoga is wonderful for prenatal conditioning, pregnant women should consult their doctors before beginning a YogaFit practice, as they would for any exercise program. Here are some key points for pregnant women to keep in mind:

- Women who are used to performing regular exercise will experience a decline in performance during pregnancy. This is unavoidable, and you should not try to compensate for it. In fact, because there's less oxygen available for aerobic exercise, you need to limit the intensity of your session and lower your target heart rate.
- Avoid overstretching. Hormonal changes cause ligaments to loosen, and going too deep into a posture can result in injury. Also avoid lower spinal twists, lunges, forward bends, and supine-lying poses, such as the Spinal Twist (seated or lying down), Warrior poses, Forward Fold (seated or standing), or Child's Pose (unless knees are apart).
- Avoid prolonged inverted postures and refrain from holding your breath because these can limit the flow of blood to the fetus. In addition, pregnancy might affect circulation, so be sure to keep warm (but overheating is also dangerous for the fetus, so dress in layers). After the first trimester, avoid prolonged periods of standing or lying flat on your back.
- Body changes remain for four to six weeks after pregnancy. New mothers should be careful not to overextend themselves. Take time to gradually work back into your regular fitness routine.

YogaFit poses can be modified to accommodate the physical changes in pregnant women's bodies. For example, in the third trimester a wall or chair can be used to aid balance. For more information on safely continuing your YogaFit practice during pregnancy and beyond, look for YogaFit's manual and DVDs for prenatal and postpartum, which can be purchased at www.yogafit.com.

Seniors

YogaFit is one of the best exercise formats for older adults, but anyone 65 and older should consult a doctor before beginning a YogaFit practice. Here are key points for seniors to keep in mind:

- YogaFit for seniors is based on simple, repetitive movements. Older yoga students can derive enormous benefits from such movements when they are combined with breathing techniques. In fact, the single most important point of focus in a YogaFit class for seniors is deep breathing.
- If you're over 65, begin each session with an extended warm-up, as we do in our YogaFit classes for seniors, and take more time to focus on

your breathing, shoulder-opening poses (such as Chest Expansion), and balance. Some poses can be done sitting in a chair, or while standing and using a chair or wall for support. At the end of your session, allow at least 10 minutes for Final Relaxation.

- The older yoga student should initially avoid certain poses, including extended periods of inversion (especially seniors with high blood pressure, glaucoma, or cataracts), extended periods of floor postures or forward flexion, and complex postures that require a lot of strength.

Again, check with your doctor about which poses are appropriate for you and when. For more information on YogaFit for seniors, look for YogaFit's manual and DVDs for seniors at www.yogafit.com.

IT'S TIME TO BEGIN

Now it's time to learn more about the YogaFit lifestyle and how to incorporate it into your life. As necessary, return to this chapter for review. The more you know about YogaFit, and the more consistently you practice, the greater the benefits you'll receive.

2

The YogaFit Lifestyle

Yoga optimizes the health of the body and mind. The word yoga means to yoke, or to bring together all aspects of the body and mind. Embracing unity and diversity, yoga's ultimate aim is a deeper connection with ourselves and the world around us. For some, this includes a deeper connection to the Divine. Once we make this connection, we can lead a life of greater joy, acceptance, and peace.

All physical yoga is hatha yoga. For many, the practice of yoga postures, or asanas, creates a desire to embrace the entire spectrum that is yoga. The YogaFit Essence, the Four Paths of Yoga, and the foundation of yoga philosophy—the Yamas and Niyamas, as described here—are a wonderful place to begin taking our yoga practice off our mats. Whether you choose to focus on asana and breathing, or to pursue study of the other various aspects of yoga as well, ultimately you will enhance your personal awareness and understanding beyond your physical body.

> YogaFit vinyasa yoga is part of the ongoing evolution of yoga in the West. Vinyasa means literally "to place in a special way," but it's also commonly called "flow" yoga because the poses move fluidly, with the breath, from one to the next. Linking the poses in this way creates strength, flexibility, endurance, and balance for greater health and mental awareness. YogaFit vinyasa yoga is highly complementary to other yoga styles with a similar focus but includes stylistic elements that make it unique.

Remember that everyone's yoga journey is different; you should feel free to pursue your yoga practice to the degree to which you are comfortable.

THE YOGAFIT ESSENCE

At YogaFit, we believe the foundation for a successful yoga lifestyle is in our ability to practice the essence of YogaFit both on and off our mats. As you read the following elements of the YogaFit Essence, consider where you might apply them to your daily life. Then, once you begin practicing the poses and workout formats, notice how they enhance your experience in the poses.

Breathing. Breathing is vitally important to your yoga practice because it gives you energy, keeps you in the moment, and facilitates the unification process of mind, body, and spirit. Breathing during your YogaFit session is typically done through the nose. Deep diaphragmatic breathing is the key to a successful practice. The breath is our most powerful tool to calm and relax our bodies and clear our minds. Effective breathing also helps us get deeper into our poses. Regardless of the pose, we always want to focus on maintaining a long, smooth breath. See chapter 3 for details on breathing techniques.

Feeling and listening to your body. In the Western world we're often disconnected from our physical bodies. Yoga can help reconnect our bodies, minds, and spirits. You want to feel something in every pose. During practice, remind yourself to check in with your body and to modify your pose to provide less or more sensation, as appropriate. When you feel something in each pose, you are grounded in the moment and aware of your body and its potential. The ability to identify and feel your feelings gives you tremendous opportunity to connect with yourself and with others honestly.

Letting go of expectations. Too often in life we have unrealistic expectations of ourselves and others. This might manifest in your yoga practice and lead to injury on the mat. Be patient with your practice, respect the process, and go at your own pace.

Letting go of competition. The great yoga philosopher Krishnamurti has said, "When you compare, you are disappointed." Your practice is your own; no two bodies are alike, and no two lives are alike. Comparison makes you feel either superior or inferior. Neither is beneficial.

Letting go of judgment. It's not your place to judge others' lifestyles or actions. Practice replacing judgment with compassion. Do you want to be judged by others for the way you look, for the way you are? Think of how unfairly you feel treated when someone who barely knows you misjudges you. The truth is most judgments are based on inadequate information. Ask yourself how much you know about a person you have placed a judgment on. Ask yourself why you feel compelled to make a judgment. Is it to make yourself feel better?

Staying present in the moment. In his book *The Power of Now*, Ekhart Tolle argues that true peace can be found only in the present moment.

He says that the present moment is the only moment in which we can truly live our lives. When you're stuck in the past or projecting into the future, you miss out on what's in front of you. On your mat, notice when your mind slips into thoughts of the past or future. If it does, simply bring your awareness back to your breath and your body.

THE PHILOSOPHY OF YOGA

Yoga is a path with a rich philosophy, and the path is open to everyone. Integral to this philosophy are the Yamas and Niyamas, or the 10 guidelines for leading a happier, healthier, and more conscious life. Many people look to the Yamas and Niyamas as a simple and appropriate way to live their lives in today's world. In times of stress or conflict, they are powerful tools to help us maintain balance and connection with a power greater than ourselves.

> As my yoga practice progressed, I noticed that I naturally desired a deeper level of understanding of the various aspects that comprise yoga. I became the witness to myself, my actions, and the ripple effect every action created. I started to desire less—less clutter, food, stimulants and depressants, possessions, mental chatter, drama, confusion, and empty conversation. I craved more peace and calm—more harmony, tranquility, simplicity, natural beauty, truth, and space. Now when faced with a conflict, crisis, challenge, decision, or fork in the road, I refer to the Yamas and Niyamas to help guide and inspire me.

Yamas

The Yamas are guidelines for how we interact with each other and the outer world. They are social disciplines to guide us in our relationships with others. The Yamas are Ahimsa, Satya, Asteya, Brahmacharya, and Aparigraha.

Ahimsa

Ahimsa is the practice of nonviolence toward yourself and other living beings in your actions, thoughts, and speech. Not only do you cause no harm, you do not accept or allow anything that causes harm. Because violence arises out of fear, anger, restlessness, and selfishness, Ahimsa advocates kindness, compassion, love, patience, self-love, and worthiness.

YogaFit Essence: Listen to your body and even your inner dialogue (self-talk) to help you in your yoga practice.

Satya

Satya is truthfulness in speech, thoughts, and deeds. To practice Satya is to exhibit honesty (with the intention of helping, not harming) while owning your feelings, valuing genuine and gentle communication, giving constructive feedback, forgiving and letting go of judgment, and taking off your "mask."

YogaFit Essence: Go at your own pace; be honest about what that pace is.

Asteya

Asteya embodies taking only what belongs to you. The guidelines for Asteya include not stealing, not coveting, and not being jealous. Practice Asteya by using objects the right way, managing your time, cultivating a sense of completeness and self-sufficiency, and letting go of your cravings.

YogaFit Essence: Let go of competition and judgment. When you stop comparing, you let go of jealousy.

Brahmacharya

Brahmacharya is moderation in all things on all levels. The guidelines for Brahmacharya include channeling your emotions, practicing self-containment, not overindulging your mind, speech, or body, and tempering your use of sex, food, and all aspects of daily life, including the environment. To practice Brahmacharya is not to be repressed but rather to control sensual cravings.

YogaFit Essence: Feel and listen to your body; when you're truly connected you'll rarely overindulge.

Aparigraha

Aparigraha is letting go of reliance on possessions and relationships, or "attachments," for your peace and happiness. When you let go of your "stuff" and your "stories," you face yourself. Letting go is not always comfortable, but it's always invigorating. Attachments can also be to food, jobs, even identities. These things in and of themselves aren't bad, but if you rely too much on your attachments you stifle your room for growth. To practice Aparigraha is to simplify—to distinguish needs from wants, to consume less and live more.

YogaFit Essence: Let go of expectations. When you refrain from excess expectations, you no longer desire to fill yourself with ultimately unfulfilling possessions, addictions, and distractions.

> Our yoga practice should teach us compassion, love, acceptance, and a desire to honor all living creatures.

Niyamas

The Niyamas are guidelines for how we interact with ourselves and our internal world. The practice of the Niyamas harnesses the energy generated from our practice and cultivation of the Yamas. Niyamas are about self-regulation, helping us maintain a positive environment in which to grow. The five Niyamas are Shaucha, Santosha, Tapas, Swadhyaya, and Ishwara-Pranidhana.

Shaucha

Shaucha is external as well as internal purity. To practice Shaucha is to clear your mind and body of toxins and negative energy, to exhibit evenness of mind, thoughts, and speech, and to practice discrimination. You do this through good health habits, including eating a clean, organic diet, living in a clear and orderly environment, using cruelty-free products, and refraining from excessive amounts of stimulants and depressants, including prescription drugs, coffee, alcohol, and processed foods.

YogaFit Essence: When you practice yoga breathing (pranayama), you cleanse your body and mind of toxins.

Santosha

Santosha invites us to maintain equanimity, or evenness of mind, through all that life offers. The guidelines for Santosha include contentment, accepting what is, and making the best out of everything. To practice Santosha is to exhibit gratitude and joyfulness, remain calm with success or failure, let go of attachment to any external status, remain focused in the face of adversity, and choose love over fear. In *The Power of Now,* Ekhart Tolle explains that when faced with a challenging situation you can choose removal, change, or acceptance. You get to decide how to find contentment.

Yogafit Essence: Be present in the moment, accepting with contentment that which you are immersed in at any given moment; live in a state of flow.

Tapas

Tapas means "heat" or "fire" and is the practice of both mental and physical discipline. The guidelines for Tapas are austerity, sacrifice, and enthusiasm for the spiritual path, regardless how difficult, and a willingness to do what is necessary to reach a goal with discipline. To practice Tapas is to exhibit determination in pursuing daily practices and your life's mission, while remaining joyful in the knowledge that outer discipline will lead to inner discipline.

YogaFit Essence: Stay in the present moment regardless how uncomfortable it becomes. Go through the heat and accept it, inviting it in. The fire brings transformation.

Swadhyaya

Swadhyaya is the practice of self-observation. It gives you a pause between stimulus and response, allowing you room to breathe, relax, feel, watch, and allow. Matters you are pondering might become clear to you in an almost organic manner, or they might take time for truth to emerge. Be open and cultivate the spirit of exploration within you. The guidelines of Swadhyaya are self-education and study. To practice Swadhyaya is not to become self-absorbed but to exhibit reflection, meditation, and a desire to know the truth.

YogaFit Essence: Let go of expectations of yourself to allow yourself to observe speech, thoughts, and actions honestly, without judgment. This leads to acceptance—and with acceptance, growth.

Ishwara-Pranidhana

The guidelines of Ishwara-Pranidhana are surrendering to God or to the light and energy of the universe. To practice Ishwara-Pranidhana is to exhibit faith, dedication, sincerity, and patience to transcend the ego, which is so resistant to surrender. Ishwara-Pranidhana is about your relationship to the divine energy of the universe. Your divine relationship might manifest in many ways, such as chanting, painting, being in nature or with animals, listening to music, or writing a poem. Everyone has a way to surrender to spirit and celebrate the universal connection.

YogaFit Essence: When you let go of judgment, you let go of trying to control. Only then can you overcome your ego and celebrate connection to that which is beyond you.

THE FOUR PATHS OF YOGA

Practicing the YogaFit Essence and the Yamas and Niyamas can guide you in living a yogic life both on and off your mat, but many people also choose to deepen their practice and foster growth by following one of the four yoga paths. While your unique personality will dictate which path or paths you are most inclined to pursue on your journey, all paths lead to greater wisdom, connection, and, eventually, the ability to surrender. The four paths are karma yoga, jnana yoga, raja yoga, and bhakti yoga.

1. *Karma yoga*

   Karma yoga is the realization of the Divine through works and duty. Karma yoga is also the basis for YogaFit's mission. This is the path of selfless service and giving. Practice karma yoga by giving back wherever you feel called, whether it's caring for friends and family, volunteering for charities and other service work, or as a YogaFit instructor teaching community service classes.

2. *Jnana yoga*

   Jnana yoga is the realization of the Divine through the acquisition of knowledge. This is the path of pursuing wisdom and intellect. Those who prefer to seek understanding through studying the words and wisdom of others are drawn to this path. If you love to study, find the texts and teachers that speak to your heart.

3. *Raja yoga*

   Raja yoga is the realization of the Divine through control of the mind and the practice of listening. This is the path of meditation. Because the yoga postures were originally created to help you quiet your mind and body for meditation, hatha yoga is included in this path. For many, the answers come only through practicing stillness.

4. *Bhakti yoga*

   Bhakti yoga is the realization of the Divine through a devotion to and love of a personal God. This is the path of love and worship. Regardless of where and how you choose to worship, practicing bhakti yoga involves focusing your heart and your efforts on the Divine.

Remember that no one path is better than another. Ultimately, they all lead to that place of Ishwara-Pranidhana, or surrender.

YOUR PATH

How you interpret these elements of yoga practice is subjective, and they often change as you grow. Yoga is not a religion, nor is it intended to conflict with anyone's culture or belief system. Rather, yoga is a way to dissolve barriers and engender a deeper connection between ourselves and others, and between ourselves and the universal spirit.

So take what you like and leave the rest. For these concepts to have a positive impact on your life, you must be prepared to hear the truth that is spoken to your heart, and to apply it. It takes work to live our truth (Tapas), but the rewards are immediate. YogaFit is a workout, yes, but it is so much more. A fit body certainly improves our quality of life, but true peace and joy are found when our bodies, minds, and spirits are strong and healthy. Be patient with yourself during the process. Growth takes time, but once it has begun, it never stops. Embrace your journey.

3

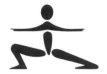

YogaFit Breathing

Breath is life. Yogis have known the amazing benefits of breathing practices for thousands of years, but scientists in the Western world have only recently established a clear connection between deep, controlled breathing and improved health. One of the greatest health benefits in our culture is stress reduction. We know that stress is linked to a number of health conditions, including high blood pressure, heart disease, and depression. Just learning how to breathe deeply, on and off the mat, can reduce, or even eliminate, many of the symptoms triggered by stress.

In traditional yoga, the breath is known as *prana*, or the universal life-force energy within all of us. Thus, your pranic body is your vital body, also known as your energy body. Classic yoga breathing techniques then are known as *pranayama*, or practices created to control the breath and harness the prana within and surrounding your body in order to create a state of inner peace. Your pranic energy corresponds to the left and right side of your body. Your right side is associated with increased energy, heat, and alertness. Your left side is associated with internal awareness, cooling, and calm. More than breath control exercises, then, pranayama is about controlling the life force. Ancient yogis, who understood the essence of prana, studied pranayama and devised methods and practices to master it—many of which YogaFit teaches and we provide here.

YogaFit breathing and pranayama techniques offer other benefits as well:

- Increased strength and control of the diaphragm (primary breathing muscle) and other core muscles.
- Increased heat and energy.
- Heightened awareness, concentration, and control.

- Increased control of prana for physical and mental balance.
- Decreased anxiety.
- Deep relaxation for the body and mind.

Once you begin to practice deep breathing regularly, you'll experience for yourself the profound impact your breath has on your mental and physical energy, and on your well-being.

> It's common during everyday life to use only the upper third of our lungs. This kind of shallow breathing is generally caused by tension or stress. Because the blood vessels are more plentiful in the lower lobes of the lungs, we need to use our entire lung capacity to get enough oxygen into our bodies, and to release the toxins eliminated as we exhale. The increased oxygen we breathe in gives us more physical energy and improves our concentration and mental clarity, which is one of the first things we lose when we're under stress. Let's focus on deep naval breathing.

THE YOGAFIT BREATH

The breathing techniques described in this chapter are essential to the YogaFit style. You'll use them in every YogaFit session for the most powerful and effective mental and physical experience.

Nose Breathing

Traditional yoga breathing practices are done exclusively through the nose. YogaFit teaches nose breathing as well because breaths taken in through your nose warm and filter the air coming into your body. These breaths keep your body warmer while you work out, which is necessary for your muscles and connective tissue to stretch safely and effectively. Breathing through your nose also demands greater concentration, which helps you stay focused and connected with your body during even the most challenging phases of your practice. Finally, nose breathing is more efficient for your heart and lungs, which is why many professional athletes practice this technique.

Exercise

Each of the following breathing practices rely on nose breathing. Practice by sitting tall, either while cross-legged on the floor or in a chair, or by lying on your back. Close your lips and breathe deeply through your nose. What do you notice about the quality of your breath? How does nose breathing make you feel?

In YogaFit, when moving from one pose to the next, you match the flow of the poses to the pace of your deepest breath. This flowing style of yoga is also known as *vinyasa*, which means "to place in special way." Although you often hold certain poses and breathe through them, at no point do you move without breathing. It's important to remember to find your own perfect pace, and to trust that with practice your breath and movement will synchronize effortlessly, making both easier.

Ujjayi Breath

Like nose breathing, you'll use *Ujjayi* breath in every YogaFit session. The only time you won't use Ujjayi breath is in the Final Relaxation pose. This technique is also used in conjunction with other pranayama techniques, as we'll describe. The purpose of Ujjayi is to make your breath barely audible, just loud enough for you alone to hear. This allows you to monitor both the quality and quantity of your breath as you work out. If you can hear your breath, you'll recognize when it's becoming rapid and shallow, or if it's staying steady and deep. Ujjayi also gives you a focal point when your mind begins to wander.

Ujjayi breathing requires you to partially close your glottis (the part in your throat that closes when you swallow but is open when you breath). Breathing this way creates a whispery sound, which is why the technique is also known as Whisper breath. Ujjayi breathing can be compared to the sound Darth Vadar makes in *Star Wars,* though not quite as amplified.

Exercise

Practice by sitting tall, either cross-legged on the floor or in a chair, or by lying on your back. Close your lips and breathe deeply through your nose. Begin Ujjayi breathing, focusing on matching the quality and quantity of every inhale to every exhale. Once you have mastered this technique at rest, try it when under stress or exertion, such as when driving in traffic or riding your bicycle.

Three-Part Breath

The Three-Part breath, also known as the Complete breath, is the simplest and most rewarding of all yogic breathing exercises. It is both purifying and energizing, and, if done slowly and evenly, can produce a sense of serenity and balance. As mentioned, in daily life, we often breathe with only the top portion of our lungs, neglecting to get the oxygen we need to function at our potential. Thus, breathing in and out at full capacity even just a few times can markedly increase blood oxygen levels and decrease carbon dioxide. Three-Part breaths are great for heightening your awareness of your breathing from moment to moment and helping you recognize, and use, the potential depth of your lungs.

In a Three-Part breath you use your diaphragm to fill your lungs completely from bottom to top. To practice this technique, first focus on expanding your belly, then your ribs, and then your chest, before exhaling completely. Three-Part breaths can be used at any time in a YogaFit session, including at the beginning and end of your session with Relaxation breath, as discussed next. Three-Part breathing is usually coupled with Ujjayi breathing for greater awareness and control.

Exercise

Sit tall and inhale, bringing your breath deep into your abdomen, then ribcage, and finally into your chest and throat. Exhale completely, letting everything go. Repeat several times.

Relaxation Breath

Relaxation breath is a slow-paced technique used to induce a state of deep relaxation and centeredness. It's the simplest and easiest method of breathing, and one we all should practice under the pressure and rush of daily life because it helps reverse the physiological symptoms of stress, including lowering the heart rate and decreasing blood pressure. Although a Relaxation breath is not as deep as a Three-Part breath, this technique also focuses on matching the length and depth of the inhale to that of the exhale. Use Relaxation breathing during the first pose of your warm-up and in your Final Relaxation pose to achieve a serene, restorative state.

Exercise

Lying comfortably on your back, relax completely. Place your right hand on your chest and your left hand on the upper part of your abdomen. Breathe so only your left hand rises during the inhale and falls during the exhale. Your right hand remains virtually motionless. Give an equal amount of time to the inhale and the exhale. Breathing this way should never be a struggle. Do only what you're able to do calmly and comfortably.

Sinking Breath

We know that trying to force flexibility causes our muscles to resist and shorten. Sinking breath is a technique that uses longer exhalations to move you gently into a deeper stretch. By extending your exhale in poses that move toward the center of the earth (Standing Forward Fold, p. 106; Downward-Facing Dog, p. 108; or Pyramid, p. 114), your muscles relax, release, and lengthen.

Exercise

Assume a relaxed pose, inhale, and feel your body lift slightly. Exhale slowly and completely, allowing your body to sink more deeply into the pose. Repeat for the length of your pose (see chapter 4).

Expanding Breath

Expanding breath is a technique focused on your inhalations and is used in poses that open your chest to the sky (Standing Backbend, p. 130; Camel, p. 134; Bridge, p. 140; or Triangle, p. 82). On every inhale you breathe in deeply, lifting and expanding your chest; you then maintain that expansiveness as you exhale. An open chest allows you to breathe more deeply. The effort required to hold your chest open builds strength and support in and around your spine.

Exercise

Assume a relaxed pose and inhale, filling your lungs deeply with air. As your chest expands, be aware of how your whole body lifts and opens as you take this breath. Keep that open feeling even while you exhale. Repeat for the length of your pose (see chapter 4).

YOGAFIT PRANAYAMA

The following pranayama techniques are used for different purposes. Review them carefully, and then incorporate those that will be of most benefit to you day to day, practice to practice. Whether or not you choose to use these techniques, remember that when it comes to breathing, if you are breathing consciously, you are doing yoga.

Alternate Nostril Breathing

Alternate Nostril breathing energetically balances your body and mind, as well as your prana, through regulation of your breath through each nostril. This is an excellent technique to center yourself at the beginning of your YogaFit session, or to help you transition into your Final Relaxation pose at the end of your practice. Many people use Alternate Nostril breathing to prepare for meditation.

Effects
- Balances your pranic (energy) body. Whether you are anxious and distracted or lethargic and fatigued (or anywhere in between), this technique helps you feel balanced. When your pranic body is balanced, you are energetic and alert, yet calm and peaceful.
- Centers you.
- Prepares you for meditation.

Restrictions

- Avoid loud or forced breathing.

Exercise

Assume the Mountain Pose (p. 66), or sit cross-legged in a comfortable position. Start by noticing the current flow of your breath. When comfortable, curl your right hand into your palm, keeping your thumb, ring finger, and pinkie extended (A). Move your right thumb to the bridge of your right nostril (B). Inhale through your left nostril. At the top of your inhale, close your left nostril with your right ring finger (while releasing your thumb) and exhale through your right nostril (C). Now inhale through your right nostril. At the top of your inhale, close your right nostril and exhale through your left nostril (D). Continue alternating at the top of each inhale. Repeat for 5 to 10 rounds. After your last exhale, unblock your nostrils and take three deep, even breaths through your nose.

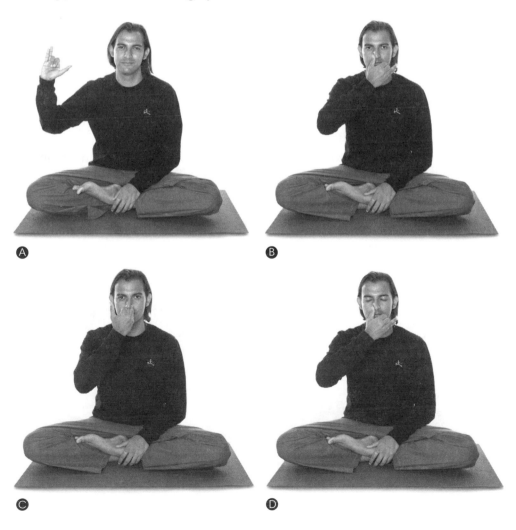

A B

C D

Single Nostril Breathing

Single Nostril breathing regulates your breathing through one nostril or the other, for either increased or decreased prana. You increase your physical and mental energy when lethargic or depressed, or decrease it if anxious or stressed. This technique also prepares you for meditation.

Following are two Single Nostril breathing techniques to balance your mind, body, and spirit. Use them in Mountains I and III (warm-up and cool-down).

Warming Single Nostril Breath

Use this technique to wake you up and warm you up. Inhaling through your right nostril activates your pranic (energy) body and increases heat, energy, and alertness.

Effects

- Energizes you.
- Activates the right side of your pranic system.

Restriction

- Avoid loud or forced breathing.

Exercise

Assume the Mountain Pose (p. 66), or sit comfortably in a cross-legged position. Start by noticing the current flow of your breath. When comfortable, curl your right hand into your palm, keeping your thumb, ring finger, and pinkie extended, as shown in figure A. Now move your right ring finger to the bridge of your left nostril (A). Close your left nostril by gently pressing your ring finger against your nose so that you're inhaling exclusively through your right nostril (B). Now close your right nostril with your right thumb,

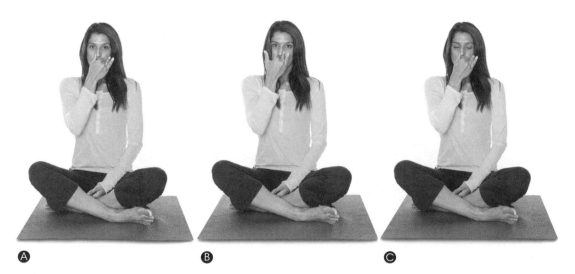

Ⓐ   Ⓑ   Ⓒ

and exhale through only your left nostril (C). Continue this pattern 5 to 10 rounds, always breathing in only through your right nostril and exhaling through your left. After your last exhale, unblock your nostrils and take three deep, even breaths.

Cooling Single Nostril Breath

Use this technique to calm down and cool down. Inhaling through your left nostril calms your pranic (energy) body to promote relaxation and centering.

Effects

- Calms you.
- Activates the left side of your pranic system.

Restriction

- Avoid loud or forced breathing.

Exercise

Assume the Mountain Pose (p. 66), or sit comfortably in a cross-legged position. Start by noticing the current flow of your breath. When comfortable, curl your right hand into your palm, keeping your thumb, ring finger, and pinkie extended, as shown in figure A on page 26. Now move your right thumb to the bridge of your right nostril (A) and inhale through your left nostril. Then close your left nostril with your right ring finger and exhale through your right nostril (B). Repeat this pattern 5 to 10 rounds, always breathing in only through your left nostril and exhaling through your right. After your last exhale, unblock your nostrils and take three deep, even breaths.

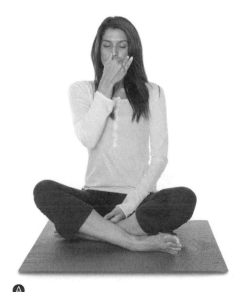

Ⓐ

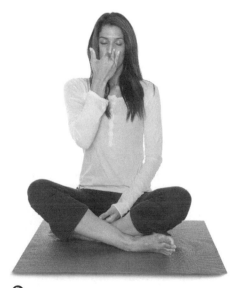

Ⓑ

Breath of Fire

The Breath of Fire uses deep, rapid breath cycles to warm your body and increase your energy. Traditionally, the Breath of Fire is not a pranayama technique but rather a *kriya*, or cleansing, practice. Many of the toxins in your body are released during your exhale, which is the focus here. Practice it during Mountains I and III (warm-up and cool-down).

Effects

- Energizes and activates the right side of your pranic system.
- Stimulates your nervous system.
- Cleanses your respiratory system.

Restrictions

- Avoid hyperventilating by focusing on strong, quick exhalations.
- Check for dizziness (if dizzy, return to Relaxation breathing).
- If you have a heart or blood pressure condition, avoid this technique.

Exercise

Assume the Mountain Pose (p. 66), or sit comfortably in a cross-legged position. Begin inhaling through your nose, keeping your mouth closed. Exhale half the air out of your lungs to a point somewhere between exhale and inhale. Your exhale should be quick and sharp, contracting your abdominal muscles. In this exercise, exhalations are short, vigorous, and active; inhalations are light and passive. Continue this rhythmic pattern for 20 to 25 breaths. Repeat two to five rounds, finishing with a deep Three-Part breath (see p. 22).

Locks

Bandha is the Sanskrit term for lock. A lock binds our physical body to our vital or energetic body. The practice of pranayama helps to harness your prana and control its flow. You can enhance this with a bandha, or a defined area within your anatomy activated through muscular contraction.

There are many locks practiced in traditional yoga, but we'll focus on two primary locks that are used in hatha yoga: root lock (*Mula Bhanda*) and belly lock (*Uddiyana Bhanda*). As you try some exercises to develop awareness, you might discover you already know how to apply a bandha.

Root Lock

Root lock is about grounding. It involves a gentle, firm contraction of the pelvic floor muscles, which activates your inner thighs and core to stabilize your pose. Root lock can also involve centering your thoughts on gaining ground and maintaining your status or standing in life. Finally, as it relates to prana, root lock is often combined with pranayama techniques.

Exercise

Root lock is the contraction of three small muscles within the perineum. Picture the base of your pelvis as a diamond, with a line drawn horizontally across the middle to create two triangles. The upper triangle is the perineum. The lower triangle is the sphincter muscle, which should remain relaxed. One way to explain root lock is comparing it to how it feels to stop your flow of urination. This is the sensation you feel when you contract your perineum.

Belly Lock

Belly lock is about creating and storing energy. It can increase your energy level, cleanse and stimulate your digestive system, and increase your lung capacity by stretching your diaphragm for deeper, more efficient breathing.

Belly lock is always combined with root lock. It involves the abdominals, diaphragm, and intercostals (muscles between the ribs). Belly lock can be performed as a core-stabilizing exercise or as a breath-holding technique. Either way, make sure you're comfortable with sustained breath retention after exhaling before performing the belly lock while holding your breath.

Exercise

Begin by inhaling to fill your lungs. Then, when exhaling, draw up and inward with your abdominal muscles to empty your lungs completely. At the end of your exhale, tuck your chin into your chest as if you were holding a small tennis ball. If practicing breath retention, hold your breath out to create a "vacuum" that draws your organs up, holding them against your diaphragm. To avoid gasping, release your abdomen and chin *before* inhaling. Practice belly lock as you perform the three following pranayama techniques and note your experience in each. Remember that belly lock builds on root lock, so contract your perineum before and during each of the exercises.

- Lying-down Three-Part breath.
- Seated Three-Part breath.
- Seated Alternate Nostril breath.

In chapter 2, you learned the YogaFit Essence and the importance of letting go when learning any aspect of yoga. This applies to the poses as well as the breath. While breathing practices are about controlling our prana, they are only effective when approached without expectations, competition, and judgment. Stay in the present, embrace the process of taking in and letting out each breath, and delight in what conscious breathing can effect in your life.

4

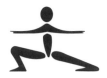

The Three Mountains of YogaFit: Warm-Up, Work, and Cool-Down

In YogaFit, we apply modern exercise science to the ancient mind–body practice of yoga. Although yoga can have a profound impact on the physical, emotional, and spiritual health of students, improper sequencing and pacing creates opportunities for physical discomfort and injury. For this reason, YogaFit classes follow a format called the YogaFit Three Mountains, a format consistent with current group exercise standards and guidelines for the safest, most effective, and consistent progression possible.

In fitness, every workout begins by preparing your body in two ways. First, you create heat by working your largest muscle groups first. This allows your muscles and connective tissue to later stretch safely, without injury (see chapter 9 for details on safe stretching and flexibility). Second, you move your muscles and joints through a comfortable range of motion, which prepares your body for more intense strength work and stretching while increasing muscular endurance. In Mountain I of a YogaFit class, you follow these guidelines by moving, or flowing, in and out of the poses continuously to build heat while introducing your muscles and joints gently to the positions you hold in Mountain II.

> *Your range of motion involves more than your muscles. Your genetic bone structure and the health of your joints also determine how flexible you are or can become. To avoid injury and get the most out of your yoga practice, relax and move only as far as you are comfortable, and match your breath with your movement.*

After your warm-up (Mountain I), your focus turns to strength, endurance, flexibility, and balance. According to fitness guidelines, you achieve optimal strength in two ways: by moving a muscle several times through a specific range of motion and by holding a muscle in contraction. In Mountain II, you do both. Most of the poses are held in isometric contraction to build strength, yet flows are often inserted to increase endurance (see The Flow Series later in this chapter). Further, the variety of poses YogaFit offers ensures that every major muscle is targeted in every class (and most minor muscles, too), maximizing your strength while maintaining balance.

Every workout should end with a cool-down. YogaFit's Mountain III brings you down to your mat for poses that focus on deep stretches to increase flexibility and lower your heart rate. As you work in Mountain III, you're decreasing the intensity of your workout and moving toward the final phase of any healthy fitness regime: rest and recovery.

YogaFit's Three Mountain format consists of three phases:

Mountain I: Warm-Up Phase	
Mountain II: Work Phase	
Mountain III: Cool-Down Phase	

Along with these three phases, YogaFit also includes two "valleys" that are extensions of Mountain I and Mountain II:

Valley I: Sun Salutations	
Valley II: Upright Standing Balance Poses	

The Flow Series

The Flow Series, also called the Half Series, is a dynamic flow of four poses that comprises the "bottom" half of the Sun Salutation, our Valley I series. You use this flow to help warm up your body in Mountain I and Valley I, and to retain heat in Mountain II.

In Mountain I, you begin with the modified version of this series: This version warms up the larger muscle groups in your upper body and moves your joints, including your spine, through their natural range of motion. It also prepares you for the next stage of your workout, Valley I (Sun Salutations), in which poses are added to the series and the more challenging option of coming off your knees is introduced.

In Mountain II your body is warm and prepared for the work phase of your practice. Inserting the Flow Series between your standing poses and standing pose sequences has several benefits:

- Keeps your body warm.
- Builds upper body and core strength.
- Increases endurance.
- Strengthens the cardiovascular system.
- Promotes musculoskeletal balance.

You can do the Flow Series on or off your knees, depending on your strength and ability. Both options target the same muscles. If you're a beginner, start on your knees until you have the strength to practice the series off your knees without struggling or dropping your hips and belly, such as might occur in the Plank or Crocodile. Repeat the series as often as you like in Mountain I as a warm-up, or in Mountain II between standing pose sequences (chapter 10 presents several workouts that include the Flow Series). Again, the number of repetitions is up to you, as long as you're listening to your body.

Here are the sequences for the Flow Series and for the modified Flow Series:

Modified Flow Series (kneeling)

Child's Pose
Kneeling Plank
Kneeling Crocodile
Cobra
Child's Pose

The Flow Series

Downward-Facing Dog
Plank
Crocodile
Upward-Facing Dog
Downward-Facing Dog

MOUNTAIN I: WARM-UP PHASE

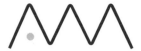

Before you begin Mountain I, the warm-up phase for YogaFit, start with three to five minutes of deep breathing (see chapter 3) to help you get centered in your body. This deep breathing oxygenates the blood, warms the body, and creates focus for your session.

After deep breathing, begin moving through one of two warm-ups (see p. 204 in chapter 10). In Mountain I, you always move, or flow, through the poses with your breath. In other words, you inhale into one pose and exhale into the next. Often you'll repeat a pose several times, using each phase of your breath to take you in and out of the posture. Movements are done through the large muscle groups (quadriceps, hamstrings, glutes, and back muscles), using the large joints of the body (knees, shoulders, hips, elbows, and spine). These movements help to warm your body, increase heart rate, and promote muscular elasticity. If you're sweating during this phase, that's a good thing.

VALLEY I: SUN SALUTATIONS

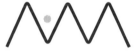

In yoga, a salutation is a series of poses with a specific focus or purpose. In YogaFit, the Sun Salutations complete your warm-up phase by working all major muscles and joints through a greater range of motion. Sun Salutations flow one breath per movement so that heat continues to build as you prepare for Mountain II.

Sun Salutations are sequential and always flow in the same order. In Valley I, the sequence is repeated on the right and left sides of the body at least twice. Remember that Sun Salutations can be modified by using the kneeling version, or the modified Flow Series.

- Mountain (*inhale*)
- Standing Forward Fold (*exhale*)
- Crescent Lunge or Kneeling Lunge (*inhale*)
- Downward-Facing Dog or Child's Pose (*exhale*)
- Plank or Kneeling Plank (*inhale*)
- Crocodile or Kneeling Crocodile (*exhale*)
- Upward-Facing Dog or Cobra (*inhale*)
- Downward-Facing Dog or Child's Pose (*exhale*)

- Crescent Lunge or Kneeling Lunge (*inhale*)
- Standing Forward Fold (*exhale*)
- Mountain Pose (*inhale*)
- Chair (*exhale*)

MOUNTAIN II: WORK PHASE

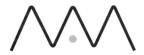

Mountain II poses are listed in the Pose Index on page 274 and also in the workouts in chapter 10. Mountain II is the work phase of your YogaFit session. In this phase you can use the heat built in Mountain I and Valley I to work into standing poses that build strength, endurance, and flexibility for the upper and lower body. Poses in Mountain II use lunging positions to build strength and flexibility in the lower body, and arm and torso positions for strength and flexibility in the upper body. Because your muscles are warm, they are now responsive to this type of movement.

Holding poses for three to five breaths on each side in Mountain II helps strengthen the muscles through isometric contraction, or through engaging a muscle or muscle group while holding it in one position. As the postures become more challenging, use Three-Part breath (p. 22) to aid concentration and provide energy. Always take a break when you need one.

VALLEY II: UPRIGHT STANDING BALANCE POSES

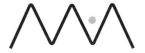

Valley II poses are listed in the Pose Index (p. 274) and also in chapter 6. In Valley II, standing balance poses are practiced with the head above the heart. Performing these poses at this point has two primary benefits: first, to improve overall balance and muscular coordination and, second, to allow your blood pressure to equalize in the upper and lower halves of your body. Equalizing your blood pressure before coming down to the floor will prevent a drop in blood pressure that could lead to dizziness, or even fainting.

Poses in Valley II are held for 5 to 10 breaths on each side. Practice as many as you like in any order that you choose.

MOUNTAIN III: COOL-DOWN PHASE

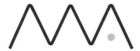

Mountain III poses are listed in the Pose Index and also in the workouts in chapter 10. Mountain III is the cool-down phase of your YogaFit session. In this phase, you use the heat created in Mountain II to move deeper into prone (on your belly), seated, and supine (on your back) poses to build strength and flexibility through deep stretching. Seated and prone poses are usually reserved for Mountain III for the sake of flow. While some Mountain III poses build strength, most offer opportunities for deep stretching and release.

To build flexibility, hold Mountain III poses for 5 to 10 breaths on each side. Holding poses for at least 30 to 45 seconds allows muscles to retain length and promotes release of muscle tension.

Note that every YogaFit session ends with 6 to 10 minutes in the Final Relaxation pose, during which you begin to physically and mentally integrate the benefits of your workout. This final phase provides an important transition from your practice back into your daily routine. See page 196 for more information on the Final Relaxation pose and its benefits.

> Scientific research shows that deep breathing and the stress-reduction benefits of the Final Relaxation phase are crucial health benefits of yoga. Because stress and stress-related conditions and illnesses are so prevalent, and because people often don't take enough time to rest, this part of your session is critical for restoration and healing. Some people actually find spending time quietly in relaxation more challenging than the poses themselves. If this is true for you, you might benefit more from this phase of the session than from any other.

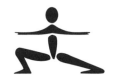

Part II

Purposeful
Poses

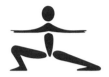

5

Core Strength and Stability

The term "core" is a buzzword in the fitness industry, and for good reason. A strong midsection, including the abs, glutes, and lower back muscles, assist us in many ways, from deep breathing to improved efficiency, balance, and athletic performance. A strong and stable center increases your energy and literally supports just about every activity you do, including getting out of bed in the morning. Conditioning your core also helps prevent back pain and injury.

Working your core does far more than just build strong muscles. When your core is strong, you *feel* strong. In other words, abdominal exercises strengthen your power center (midsection), enhancing self-esteem and boosting positive energy. A powerful midsection enhances the qualities of the third chakra, strengthening willpower, personal power, determination, and discipline (see appendix A, p. 269).

Nearly all the YogaFit poses increase core strength and stability. Whether you're standing, balancing, twisting, or inverting, you use your core to keep you steady. This chapter focuses on poses that target your midsection.

A core muscle people often neglect to target in workouts is the diaphragm, the dome-shaped muscle that separates your chest cavity and lungs from your abdominal area, where most vital organs are located. The diaphragm is your primary breathing muscle. Because your circulatory, respiratory, and nervous systems are all affected by your ability to take a deep breath, you need to regularly exercise your diaphragm. YogaFit's Three-Part breath, along with other breathing exercises described in chapter 3, target the diaphragm.

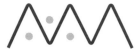

Plank and Kneeling Plank

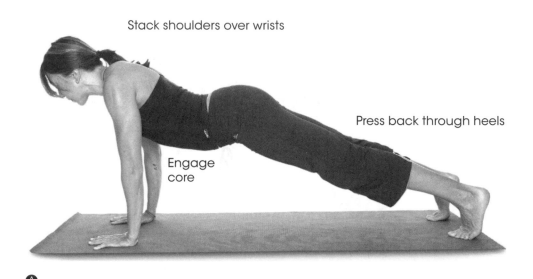

Stack shoulders over wrists

Press back through heels

Engage
core

Ⓐ

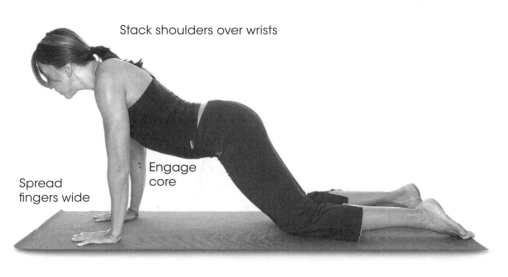

Stack shoulders over wrists

Spread
fingers wide

Engage
core

Ⓑ

On or off the knees, the Plank pose works many major muscles of the upper body and core. Use this pose in Mountains I and II and in Sun Salutations (Valley I).

▶ **Strengthens**: Abdominals • Lower Back • Chest • Shoulders • Triceps

Getting into the pose

Plank (A): From the Downward-Facing Dog, shift forward until your shoulders are directly above your wrists. Press your heels back toward the wall behind you. Reach forward through the crown of your head. Keep your back straight and abdominals firm.

Kneeling Plank (B): From the Child's Pose, shift forward until your shoulders are directly above your wrists. Keep your back straight and abdominals firm.

Holding the pose

In Mountain II, you can pause and hold the Plank or Kneeling Plank pose for three to five breaths. Keep your body aligned, hips slightly elevated. In Mountain I or Valley I, move through the Plank or Kneeling Plank as part of the Flow Series or Sun Salutations.

Modification

If you're a beginner or if your midsection sags in the Plank pose, practice the Kneeling Plank.

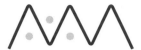

Crocodile and Kneeling Crocodile

Bend elbows back

Engage core

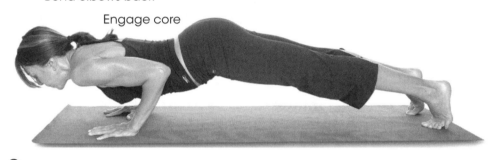

Ⓐ

Bend elbows back

Engage core

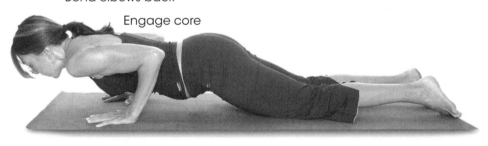

Ⓑ

Use the Crocodile after the Plank and Kneeling Plank poses to work the upper body and core in Mountains I and II, as well as in Sun Salutations (Valley I). Lower into the Crocodile as you exhale, moving right into the Cobra or the Upward-Facing Dog (pp. 44 and 46) on the next inhale.

▷ **Strengthens**: Abdominals • Lower Back • Chest • Shoulders • Triceps

Getting into the pose

Crocodile (A): From the Plank, push forward with your toes and hug your ribcage with your elbows. Lower your chest, keeping your abdominals strong and hips stationary.

Kneeling Crocodile (B): From the Kneeling Plank, shift forward, bringing your shoulders over your fingertips. Hug your ribcage with your elbows and lower your chest, keeping your abdominals strong and hips stationary.

Modification

If you're a beginner or if your midsection sags in the Crocodile pose, practice the Kneeling Crocodile.

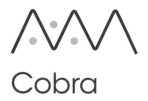

Cobra

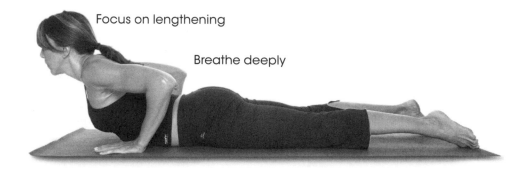

Focus on lengthening

Breathe deeply

Of all the backbending postures in yoga, the ones done on the belly are the most popular. Practice the Cobra for a strong, supple back and open chest. The Cobra follows the Kneeling Crocodile in Mountains I and II, as well as in Valley I as part of Sun Salutations. Because you're already down on the floor, you can also use the Cobra in Mountain III. Before you begin, review the introduction to chapter 7 for information on safe and effective backbending.

Strengthens: Upper Back (Rhomboids)
Stretches: Abdominals • Chest

Getting into the pose

From your belly, rest your hands lightly on the floor next to your chest. Use your back to lift your chest up and forward. Draw your shoulders back and down.

Holding the pose

Keep the back of your neck long and your lower body strong. Without pushing with your hands, lengthen your torso as you lift. In Mountain I or Valley I, move through the Cobra as part of the modified Flow Series or Sun Salutations. In Mountain II hold for 3 to 5 breaths; in Mountain III hold for 5 to 10 breaths. The challenge of lifting away from the floor against the pull of gravity is offset by the ease of exiting the backbend. Release slowly and push back to the Child's Pose (p. 164).

Upward-Facing Dog

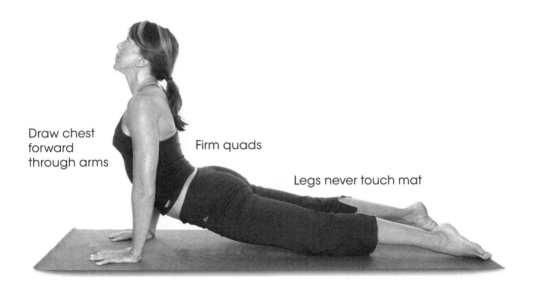

Draw chest forward through arms

Firm quads

Legs never touch mat

The Upward-Facing Dog is part of the Flow Series, but it is also a backbend. Use this pose in Mountains I and II, and in Valley I to stretch the front of your body and strengthen the muscles of your lower body and back. Before you begin, check chapter 7 for information on safe and effective backbending.

Strengthens: Glutes • Upper Back • Lower Back • Triceps
Stretches: Chest • Abdominals • Hip Flexors

Getting into the pose

From the Crocodile, place the tops of your feet on the floor and straighten your arms. Pull your chest up and forward, keeping your lower back long and your abdominals strong.

Holding the pose

In Mountain II, pause and hold the Upward-Facing Dog for three to five breaths. Continue to draw forward, engaging the muscles in your lower legs and glutes. Keep your elbows unlocked and your shoulders away from your ears. In Mountain I or Valley I, move through the Upward-Facing Dog as part of the Flow Series or Sun Salutations.

Modification

If you're healing from a wrist or lower back injury, practice the Cobra.

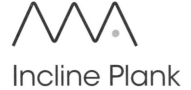

Incline Plank

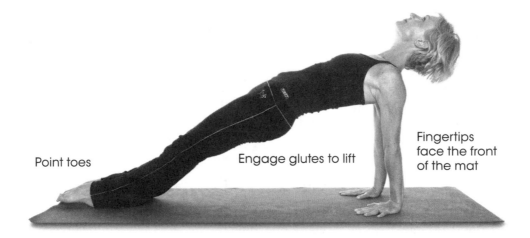

Point toes

Engage glutes to lift

Fingertips
face the front
of the mat

Use the Incline Plank in Mountain III to stretch the front of your body and build core strength in the back of your body.

Strengthens: Glutes • Shoulders • Triceps • Calves
Stretches: Chest

Getting into the pose

From a seated position, extend your legs. Place your palms on the floor behind you with fingertips spread and pointing toward your body. Press down through your hands to lift your hips toward the sky. Keeping your legs together, point your toes toward the floor. Look straight up to the sky without letting your head drop back.

Holding the pose

Engage your glutes and continue lifting your hips, keeping your body straight; maintain a slight bend in your elbows to avoid locking out your joints.

Modifications

For wrist injuries or discomfort, make "fists for wrists" with palms facing each other. If your neck fatigues, look forward rather than dropping your head back.

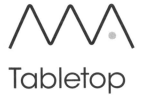

Tabletop

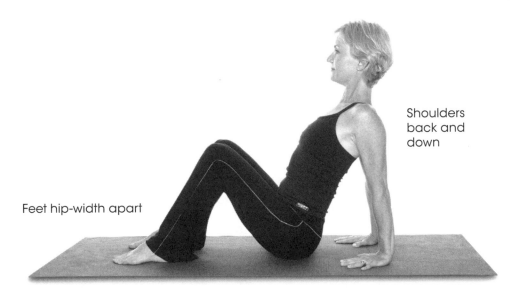

Shoulders back and down

Feet hip-width apart

A

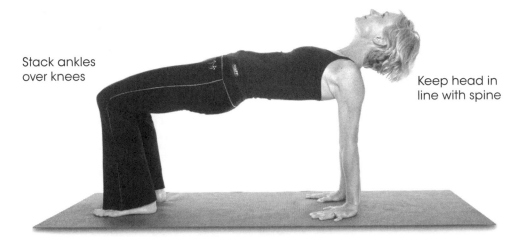

Stack ankles over knees

Keep head in line with spine

B

Use the Tabletop in Mountain III to stretch the front of your body and build core strength in the back of your body. Because your knees are bent in Tabletop, this pose requires less core strength and more shoulder flexibility than the Incline Plank. Practice both poses to maximize the benefits.

Strengthens: Glutes • Hamstrings • Shoulders • Triceps
Stretches: Chest • Hip Flexors

Getting into the pose

From a seated position, extend your legs. Place your palms on the floor behind you with fingertips spread and pointing toward your body. Place the soles of your feet flat on the floor hip-width apart (A). Press down through your hands and feet to lift your hips toward the sky (B). Look straight up to the sky without letting your head drop back.

Holding the pose

Engage your glutes and continue lifting your hips, keeping your body straight. Avoid locking your elbows.

Modifications

For wrist injuries or discomfort, make "fists for wrists" with palms facing each other. If your neck fatigues, look forward rather than dropping your head back.

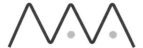

Side Plank and Kneeling Side Plank

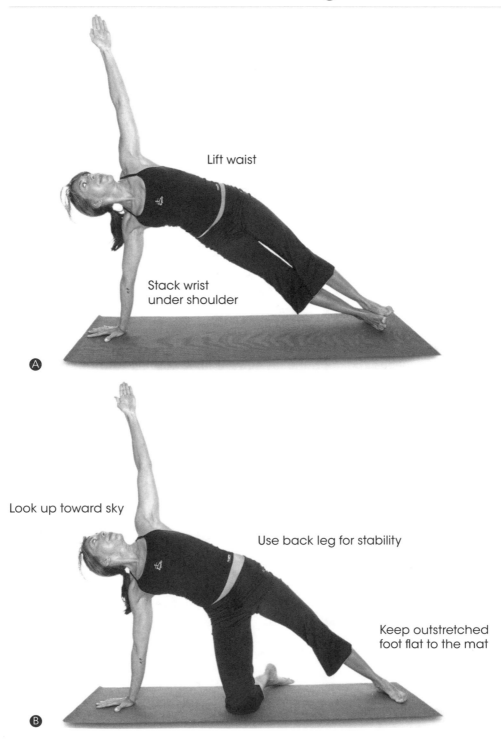

Lift waist

Stack wrist
under shoulder

(A)

Look up toward sky

Use back leg for stability

Keep outstretched
foot flat to the mat

(B)

Side Plank and Kneeling Side Plank target the obliques, the two layers of muscle in your torso that work together to help you exhale, side bend, and twist. Practice this pose in Mountain II or Mountain III, using extra caution if you're healing a shoulder.

Strengthens: Abdominals • Lower Back • Shoulders
Stretches: Obliques

Getting into the pose

Side Plank (A): Begin in the Plank pose. Inhale, reaching your arm to the sky and opening your torso to the side of your mat, keeping your wrist under your shoulder. Roll to the edges of your feet, placing your top foot on the floor behind your bottom foot. For a greater challenge, stack your feet.

Kneeling Side Plank (B): From the Plank pose, place your right knee below your hip. Move your right foot slightly to the right (like a kickstand) for stability. Straighten your left leg out as you reach your left arm to the sky. Press your left foot into the floor, pointing your toes toward the side of your mat.

Holding the pose

For the Plank and Kneeling Side Plank poses, lift the top side of your ribcage and waist toward the sky and press your hips forward. Look up at your top hand. Keep a slight bend in your elbow. Switch sides.

Modifications

If you're a beginner, practice the Kneeling Side Plank. Use extra caution if you're healing a shoulder. For wrist injuries or discomfort, make a fist instead of placing your hand flat on the floor. For knee pain or injuries, use caution and place a knee pad on the mat for comfort.

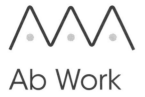

Ab Work

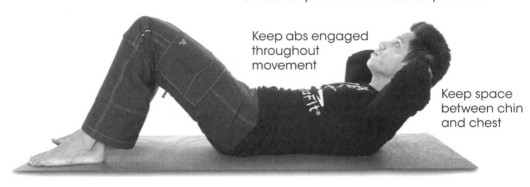

Exhale as you lift and inhale as you lower

Keep abs engaged throughout movement

Keep space between chin and chest

A

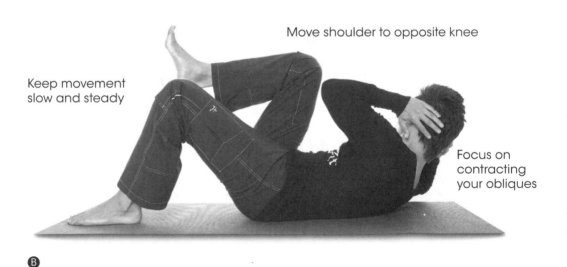

Move shoulder to opposite knee

Keep movement slow and steady

Focus on contracting your obliques

B

Abdominal exercises isolate and strengthen the muscles in your waist and abdomen. Because you do them on your back, you work against gravity to lift your body away from the floor, building strength and endurance. Be sure to release slowly back down to the floor, instead of dropping. Applying equal effort in both directions works the muscles without the benefit of momentum, for twice the strength.

When doing abdominal exercises keep space between your chin and chest to isolate your abdominals and avoid pulling on your neck. Press your lower back to the ground, keeping your stomach firm and flat. Keep your elbows back with fingers interlaced to support your head (thumbs along your neck or jaw). Exhale as you lift; inhale as you release.

In Mountain I, flow abdominal exercises with your breath for muscular endurance and heat. In Mountains II or III, flow with your breath or else hold and breathe three to five breaths to increase muscular strength.

Strengthens: Abdominals

Getting into the pose

Abdominal Curl (A): Start on your back with your feet flat on the floor and knees up. Place your hands behind your head with your fingers interlaced. As you exhale, slowly lift your head, neck, and shoulders away from the floor. Inhale and release slowly back toward the floor without ever completely relaxing your abdomen.

Yoga Bicycle (B): For oblique work, start on your back with your feet flat on the floor and knees up. Place your hands behind your head with fingers interlaced. Exhale, lifting your head, neck, and shoulders away from the floor as you bring one knee to your chest. Twist, bringing the opposite shoulder toward the opposite knee. Inhale and release slowly back toward the floor without ever completely relaxing your abdomen. For an extra challenge, extend your other leg out above the floor, pushing through the heel.

Holding the pose

In Mountains I, II, or III, flow either exercise with your breathing or, in Mountains II or III, pause at the top of the movement and breathe deeply for three to five breaths.

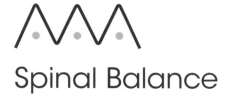

Spinal Balance

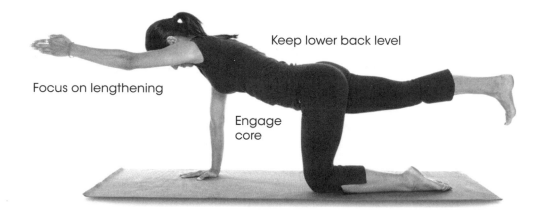

Keep lower back level

Focus on lengthening

Engage core

Part of many fitness programs, Spinal Balance improves balance and increases core strength.

> **Strengthens**: Glutes • Upper Back • Lower Back • Abdominals • Shoulders

Getting into the pose

From your hands and knees, extend one arm and the opposite leg parallel to the floor. Keeping a neutral spine, create a straight line with your arm, torso, and leg.

Holding the pose

Keep your low back level and draw your abdominals up and in. In any Mountain, focus on reaching forward through your crown and fingers and then back through your extended foot. Remember that length is more important than lift. In Mountain I, warm up your body by inhaling and lifting your opposite arm and opposite leg, releasing as you exhale and alternating sides for 5 to 10 repetitions. In Mountains II or III, hold the pose for three to five breaths, and then switch sides.

Modifications

For wrist injuries or discomfort, make "fists for wrists" with palms facing each other. Or lift just your arms or just your legs while building strength and balance. For knee pain or injuries, place a knee pad on the mat.

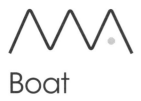

Boat

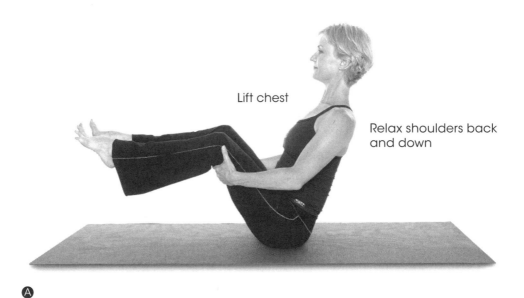

Lift chest

Relax shoulders back and down

Ⓐ

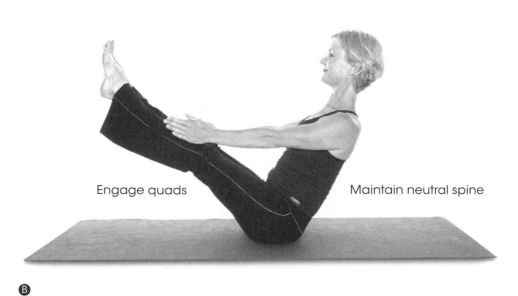

Engage quads

Maintain neutral spine

Ⓑ

Use the Boat pose in Mountain III to strengthen your core and improve your balance. Practice the Boat after the Seated Forward Fold (p. 124) to assist you in maintaining a neutral spine by lengthening your back and hamstrings.

Strengthens: Abdominals • Hip Flexors • Quads

Getting into the pose

Sitting tall on the floor, bend your knees and hold onto your hamstrings. Slowly lift one foot at a time away from the floor, keeping your back long. Reach forward with your arms as you balance on your sitting bones (A). For a greater challenge, straighten your legs and reach forward without rounding your back (B).

Holding the pose

Focus on your breath to lengthen your spine and lift your chest, relaxing your shoulders back and down.

Modification

If you're a beginner or if you have back injuries, keep your feet on the floor and continue holding onto your hamstrings.

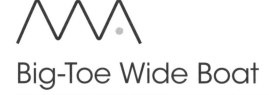

Big-Toe Wide Boat

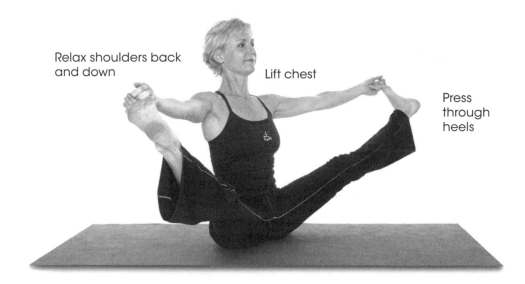

Relax shoulders back and down

Lift chest

Press through heels

This variation of the Boat pose focuses less on strength and more on stretching the legs. Use the Boat and Big-Toe Wide Boat poses in Mountain III for a well-rounded practice.

Strengthens: Upper Back • Biceps
Stretches: Hamstrings • Hip Adductors

Getting into the pose

From the Boat pose, bend your knees slightly and balance on your sitting bones. Grab your big toes with your middle and index fingers, inhale, and press through your heels to straighten your legs as far as you feel comfortable.

Holding the pose

Pull your feet back and lift your chest up and forward, finding a point of balance. Release your feet before coming down.

Modification

If you have tight hamstrings or difficulty balancing, keep your knees bent.

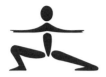

6

Standing and Balance Poses

The idea that yoga is focused entirely, or primarily, on improving flexibility is a misconception. Although yoga does work to lengthen muscles and release tightness, a more fundamental intention of yoga involves balance.

Being left- or right-handed (or footed) contributes to imbalance. We favor one side of our bodies to do everything from talking on the phone, to carrying a child on one hip, to swinging a golf club. Depending on our work or play, we tend to favor certain positions as well. Cyclists spend hours each week crouched forward in their seat, whereas others stand all day behind a cash register, often with their weight shifted to one leg. Eventually, this kind of unconscious favoritism that leads to imbalance shows up in the form of tension headaches, minor injuries, or chronic pain. The good news is that it's never too late to get back into proper alignment.

Most people spend a lot of time on their feet, but rarely do they stand at attention. Yoga teaches you to turn your awareness away from distractions and toward what's going on in your body. In this chapter you'll have the opportunity to recognize where you need to focus your efforts and then to patiently and persistently do the work of building strength, endurance, and flexibility as needed.

> Yoga teaches that when your body is balanced, your mind is balanced. When you feel good physically, you have more positive energy and fewer distractions. But to arrive at this point, you have to slow down and enjoy the process.

Standing Poses

The standing poses are used in Mountains I and II (warm-up and work phases). These are the standing poses we'll look at in this chapter:

- Mountain Pose
- Moonflowers
- Sunflowers
- Sun Pose
- Standing Lateral Flexion
- Warrior I
- Warrior II
- Reverse Warrior

- Triangle and Extended Triangle
- Side Angle and Extended Side Angle
- Bound Angle and Bound Triangle
- Chair and Balance Chair
- Warrior III
- Standing Splits
- Balancing Half-Moon

Remember that Mountain I poses move with the breath. For every inhale you move in one direction, and for every exhale you move in the opposite direction. Many Mountain I poses can also be used in Mountain II. In this case, instead of flowing with the breath, you hold the pose for three to five breaths (and, if appropriate, switch sides and repeat).

" In every standing pose you begin by bringing your awareness to your feet (SPA 1). Rather than just standing on the surface of the earth, you establish a base, which is the foundation on which you create all other actions in the pose. By standing with your feet hip-width apart and pressing down equally through the front and back halves of your feet, you activate the muscles of your legs and hips. This engages your core, gives you stability, and lets you move into another pose when you're ready. You should practice the poses barefoot. This keeps your feet strong, flexible, and healthy, preventing problems in your ankles, knees, hip, and other areas. "

Many of the standing poses are included only in Mountain II because they involve deeper stretches and greater strength. In such poses is where the real work of realigning takes place. Studies show that standing yoga poses, like the ones in this chapter, significantly increase bone density, which helps prevent osteoporosis. Men and women alike need to increase bone density as they age, and weight-bearing activities such as yoga offer excellent protection.

When practicing the standing poses, remember to do the following:

- Hold for three to five breaths.
- Practice SPA (see chapter 1).
- Focus on the part of your body in which you feel the most sensation.

- Listen to your breath. If it becomes rapid or shallow, rest or move to another pose. If it is long and deep, stay a little longer.

Standing Balance Poses

These are the standing balance poses:

- Tree
- Eagle
- Standing Balance Pigeon
- Dancer

The standing balance poses are done in Valley II, before you come down to the floor. Although many of the standing poses in yoga require balance, these poses are done on one foot to command awareness and to identify differences between left and right.

Note that Warrior III, Standing Splits, and Balancing Half-Moon, listed in the standing poses section, are also standing balance poses; however, because in each of them the head is not above the heart (necessary to equalize blood pressure), they are not considered Valley II poses. That said, they can be paired with Tree, Eagle, Standing Balance Pigeon, or Dancer because they provide all other benefits of balance work.

When practicing the standing balance poses, remember to do the following:

- Practice SPA (see chapter 1).
- Hold for 5 to 10 breaths on each side to equalize your blood pressure and improve concentration.
- Be aware of how your body feels.
- Find a focal point on the wall or floor in front of you.
- Focus on your breath. A tendency in standing balance work is to hold your breath, but if you focus on breathing the balance will come more easily.
- Relax. While working to build strength in these postures, trying too hard sometimes thwarts your efforts.

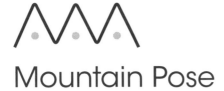

Mountain Pose

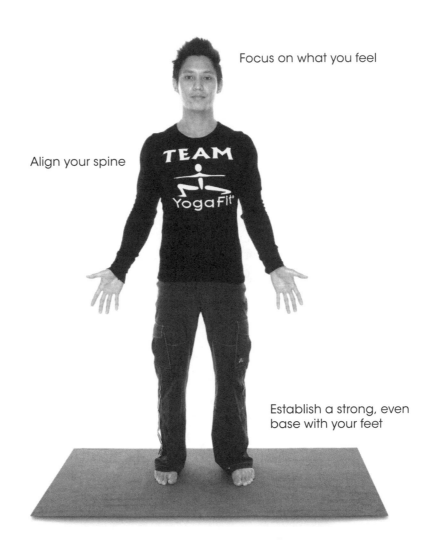

Focus on what you feel

Align your spine

Establish a strong, even base with your feet

The Mountain Pose is often where you begin your practice with three to five minutes of Three-Part breath or Relaxation breath. With your eyes open or closed, this is also a strong, steady place you can come back to at any time during your practice to become aware of how your body feels and determine if you should work harder or perhaps take a step back. Just as no two mountains are alike, no two bodies are alike. Use this pose whenever necessary to appreciate your uniqueness.

Strengthens: The mind–body connection

Getting into the pose

Stand tall at the top of your mat with arms at your sides and feet hip-width apart. Slightly bend your knees and press down through your feet. Reach down through your fingers to relax your shoulders away from your ears. Lift your chest slightly, then engage your core by firming your glutes and abdominals. Point your tailbone toward the floor.

Holding the pose

Breathe deeply into your ribcage and chest, relax your shoulders, and close your eyes, if you like.

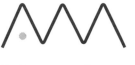

Moonflowers

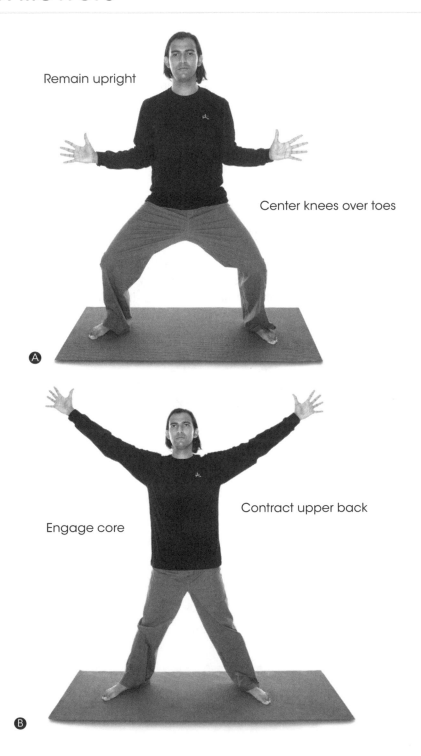

Remain upright

Center knees over toes

Ⓐ

Engage core

Contract upper back

Ⓑ

Moonflowers is a Mountain I pose. Match the pace of your movement to the pace of your breath.

> **Strengthens**: Quads • Hamstrings • Abdominals • Upper Back • Shoulders

Getting into the pose

Step back to face the long edge of your mat. Open your thighs and turn your toes out and heels in for a plié squat. Bend your elbows and place them next to your waist and point your knees straight out over your toes (A). Inhale as you straighten your arms (palms forward) and legs (B); exhale as you draw down and in. Continue to move through a comfortable range of motion as your body warms up. When ready, transition into Sunflowers or another Mountain I pose.

Modification

If you have knee concerns, come only to a comfortable place in the squat, pointing your knees over the center of your feet.

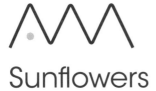

Sunflowers

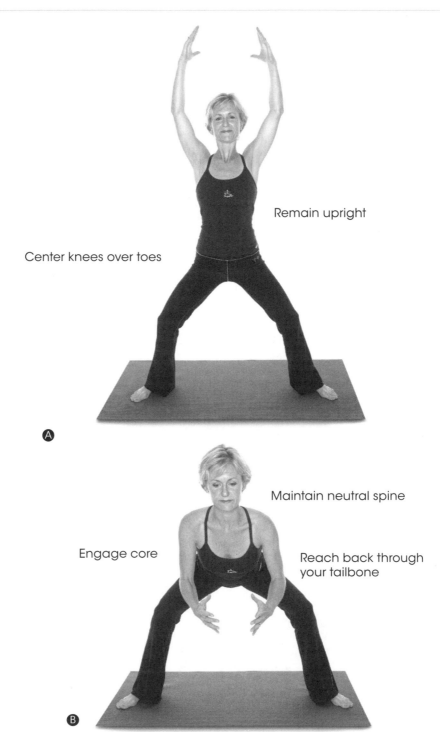

Remain upright

Center knees over toes

(A)

Maintain neutral spine

Engage core

Reach back through
your tailbone

(B)

Sunflowers builds on Moonflowers in Mountain I by working large muscle groups to build heat and moving the joints through a comfortable range of motion. Both poses prepare your body for more work and deeper stretches.

Strengthens: Quads • Hamstrings • Abdominals • Upper Back • Lower Back • Shoulders

Getting into the pose

Step back to face the long edge of your mat. As in Moonflowers, open your thighs and turn your toes out and heels in for a plié squat. Bend your elbows and place them next to your waist; point your knees straight out over your toes. Inhale as arms move overhead (A); exhale and hinge forward from the hips, reaching your tailbone back and keeping a neutral spine as you sweep your arms toward the floor (B). Inhale back to starting position. Continue to move through a comfortable range of motion as your body warms up.

Modifications

If you have knee concerns, come only to a comfortable place in the squat, pointing your knees over the center of your feet. For less intensity or shoulder concerns, place hands on thighs.

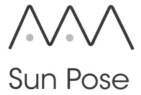

Sun Pose

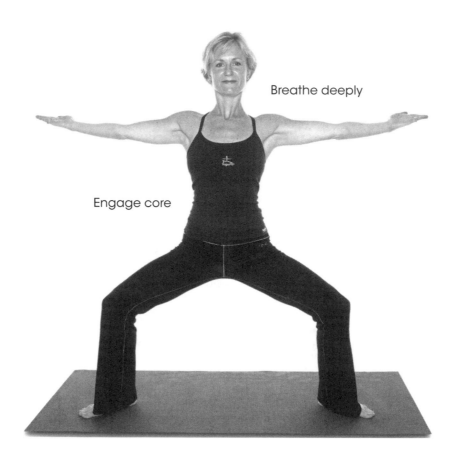

Breathe deeply

Engage core

The Sun Pose is a terrific Mountain II pose for strengthening and toning many muscles in your legs and hips. Breathe deeply to maximize the benefits. Sun Pose is also a Mountain I pose.

Strengthens: Quads • Hamstrings • Upper Back • Shoulders
Stretches: Chest

Getting into the pose

Step back to face the long edge of your mat. Open your thighs and turn your toes out and heels in for a plié squat. Extend your arms at shoulder height, palms facing up. Slowly sink your hips and hold. Squeeze your inner thighs to come back up.

Holding the pose

Make sure your weight is on your heels and your spine is straight.

Modification

If you have shoulder concerns, rest hands on hips or thighs.

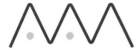

Standing Lateral Flexion

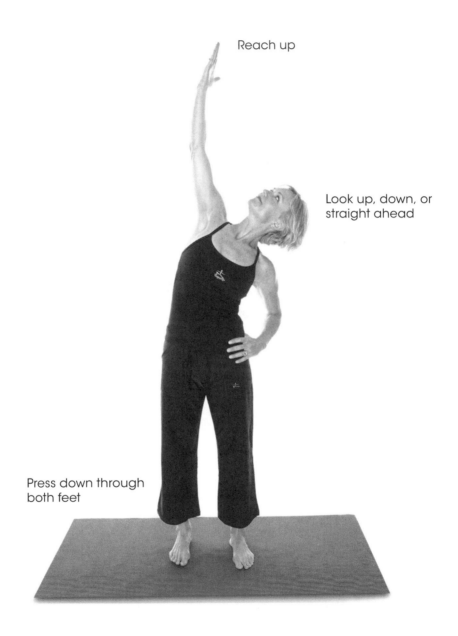

Reach up

Look up, down, or
straight ahead

Press down through
both feet

Practice this pose between standing poses to stretch and strengthen your torso. Move side to side with your breath in Mountain I, or hold for three to five breaths on each side in Mountain II.

Strengthens: Quads • Obliques • Abdominals • Shoulders
Stretches: Obliques

Getting into the pose

Lift arms over your head. Create dynamic tension by lifting your upper body and pressing down through your feet. Slide one hand down the outer thigh and reach the other hand toward the sky. Gently lean to the side without dropping your chest.

Holding the pose

In Mountain II, breathe into your sides, ribcage, waist, and chest. Keep your head in line with your spine. Don't let your upper body fall forward. Come up and switch sides.

Modification

For more lower back support, place your lower hand on your hip.

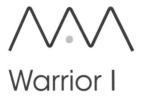

Warrior I

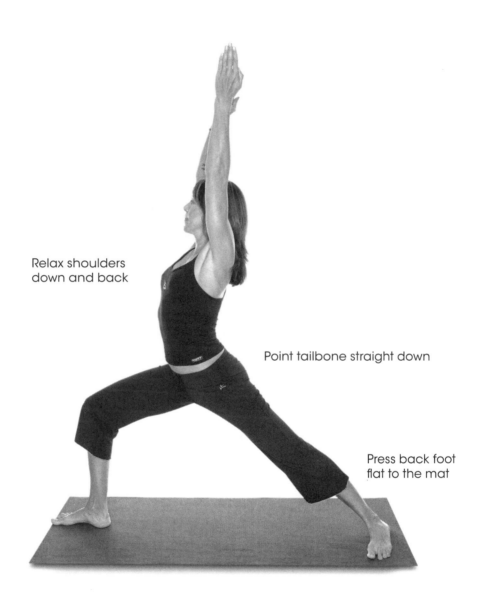

Relax shoulders
down and back

Point tailbone straight down

Press back foot
flat to the mat

This pose is part of the Warrior series. Benefits include increased physical and mental strength, enhanced power, and determination. This Mountain II pose is often repeated several times in a session followed by other standing Mountain II poses.

The Warrior poses—Warrior I, Warrior II (p. 78), Reverse Warrior (p. 80), and Warrior III (p. 90)—are primarily focused on building heat and strength. When you hold these challenging standing positions steady and breathe deeply, you also increase your ability to deal with stress. Keep in mind that aggression, however, saps your strength: A peaceful Warrior is a powerful Warrior.

Try the Warrior poses in a sequence with other standing Mountain II poses, such as Warrior I, Warrior II, Reverse Warrior, or Triangle. Do the series first on one side, then the other, doing the Flow Series (p. 32) between them. Or do the same pose once on each side before moving on. Just be sure to focus equally on the left and right for balance.

Strengthens: Quads • Hamstrings • Upper Back • Shoulders
Stretches: Hip Flexors • Hip Adductors • Calves

Getting into the pose

From the Mountain Pose, step back into a short stance and align your heels. Bend your front knee, stacking it over your ankle. Straighten your back leg, turning your toes slightly forward. Square your hips and shoulders with the front of your mat. Raise your arms to the sky.

Holding the pose

Continue to press the outer edge of your back foot into the mat. Open your hands and spread your fingers wide. Relax your shoulders and point your tailbone straight down. Engage your abdominals as you lift up with your upper body and sink into your forward leg. Keep your forward knee over your ankle. Switch sides.

Modifications

To decrease the intensity, slightly straighten your forward leg or shorten your stance, or both. For shoulder discomfort, bring your hands to a prayer position.

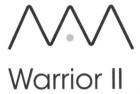

Warrior II

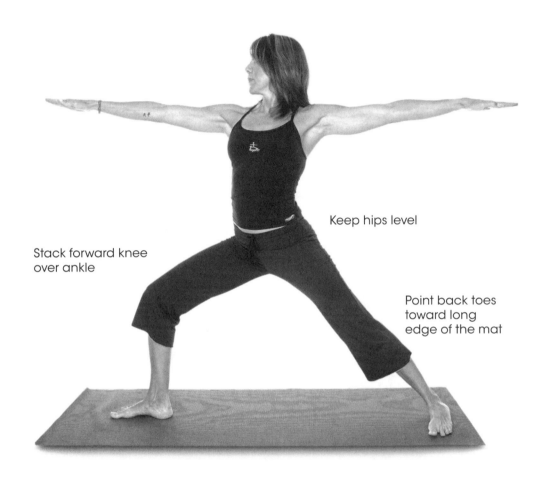

Keep hips level

Stack forward knee
over ankle

Point back toes
toward long
edge of the mat

Warrior II follows Warrior I within Mountain II. Here, for improved strength, focus, and discipline, emphasize moving energy outward while turning your awareness inward (see Warrior I on p. 76 for more information on the benefits of the Warrior poses).

Strengthens: Quads • Hamstrings • Hip Abductors • Shoulders
Stretches: Hip Adductors • Hip Flexors

Getting into the pose

From Warrior I, keep your heels aligned as you open your hips and shoulders to the long edge of your mat. Lower your arms parallel to the floor, reaching out in opposite directions through your fingers. Keep your front knee bent and hips level. Look over your front hand.

Holding the pose

Lift your upper body and reach through your fingers in opposite directions. Sink through your lower body, keeping your knee over your ankle. Engage abdominals and relax your shoulders back and down. If you feel yourself fatiguing, focus on your hands to boost your energy. Open your palms and spread your fingers wide to bring the entire pose to life.

Modifications

To decrease the intensity, slightly straighten the forward leg or shorten your stance, or both. For shoulder discomfort, bring your hands to a prayer position.

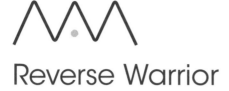

Reverse Warrior

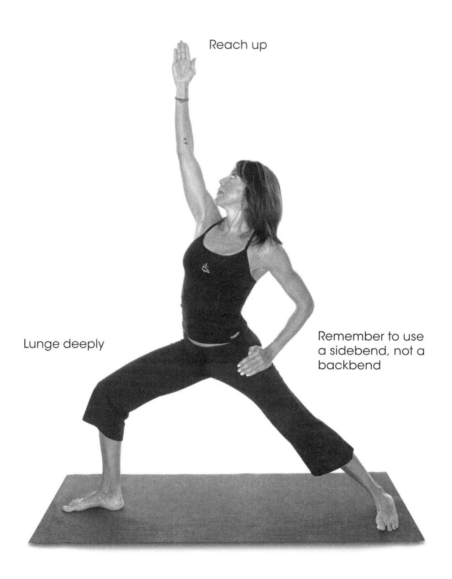

Reach up

Lunge deeply

Remember to use a sidebend, not a backbend

Practice Reverse Warrior in Mountain II to stretch and strengthen your upper and lower body (see p. 76 for the benefits of the Warrior poses).

Strengthens: Quads • Hamstrings • Lower Back • Upper Back • Abdominals • Shoulders
Stretches: Hip Flexors • Hip Adductors • Obliques

Getting into the pose

From Warrior II, keep your front knee bent and lift your forward arm toward the sky. Turn your palm toward the back of your mat. Rest your back hand lightly on your back leg. Use core strength to support a gentle side bend.

Holding the pose

Sink through your lower body while lifting up and out of your waist. Watch your knee-to-ankle alignment on your forward leg. Switch sides.

Modifications

To decrease intensity, slightly straighten your forward leg or shorten your stance, or both. For shoulder discomfort, bring your hands to a prayer position.

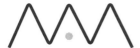

Triangle and Extended Triangle

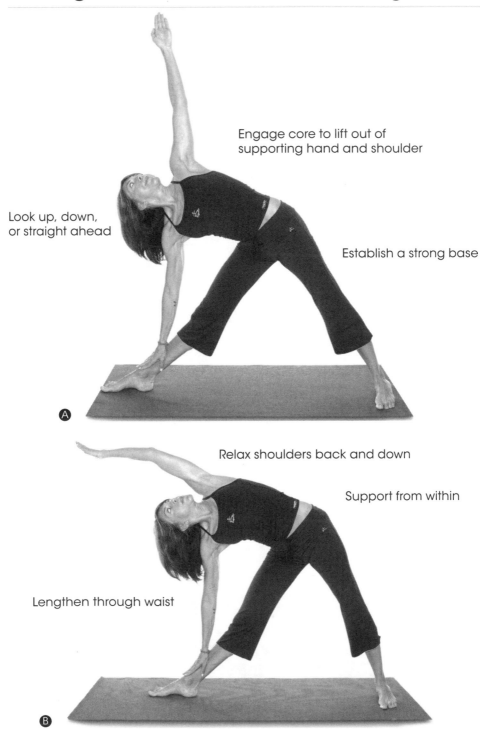

Engage core to lift out of supporting hand and shoulder

Look up, down, or straight ahead

Establish a strong base

(A)

Relax shoulders back and down

Support from within

Lengthen through waist

(B)

The Triangle Pose and Extended Triangle Pose represent a strong mental and physical foundation formed by the two bottom points of the triangle. From here, you can begin looking up to explore the third point—the spiritual. Practice these poses within Mountain II.

Strengthens: Quads • Obliques • Hip Flexors • Shoulders
Stretches: Hamstrings • Hip Adductors

Getting into the pose

Triangle (A): From Warrior II or the Side Angle pose, straighten your front leg. Reach forward and then lower your hand to your shin or ankle. Lift your back arm to the sky, opening your chest. Look up, down, or straight ahead, finding a comfortable place for your neck.

Extended Triangle (B): For an added challenge, from the Triangle, drop your top arm over your ear and roll your chest toward the sky.

Holding the pose

Press your feet away from each other, keeping a slight bend in your forward knee. Your nose stays over your leg, not in front of it. Engage your glutes. Breathe length into your spine, allowing your inner strength to fuel your outer strength. Switch sides.

Modification

If your hamstrings are tight, place your hand on a block.

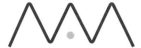

Side Angle and Extended Angle

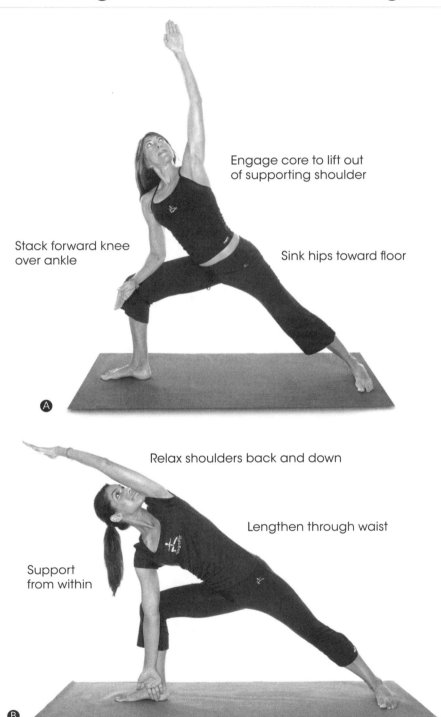

Engage core to lift out of supporting shoulder

Stack forward knee over ankle

Sink hips toward floor

Relax shoulders back and down

Lengthen through waist

Support from within

Practice the Side Angle and Extended Angle poses within Mountain II to build strength and flexibility in your legs and hips. Your obliques also get a great workout as you lengthen your spine over your forward leg and roll your chest toward the sky.

Strengthens: Quads • Obliques • Hip Flexors • Hip Abductors • Shoulders
Stretches: Hip Adductors • Calves

Getting into the pose

Side Angle (A): From a Warrior stance, bend your front knee and place your forearm on your thigh, or place your hand in front of your leg on the floor. Reach your top arm to the sky.

Extended Angle (B): For a greater challenge, from the Side Angle, lower your top arm over your ear, palm down. Reach forward through your fingertips as you push into your back foot.

Holding the pose

In either pose, rotate your chest toward the sky and press your hand into the earth. Tighten your glutes while lowering your hips and pressing them forward. With every inhale, lengthen your spine. With every exhale, sink your hips toward the floor. Switch sides.

Modification

For either version of the pose, place your bottom hand on a block to help lift and support your torso as you build core strength.

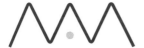

Bound Angle and Bound Triangle

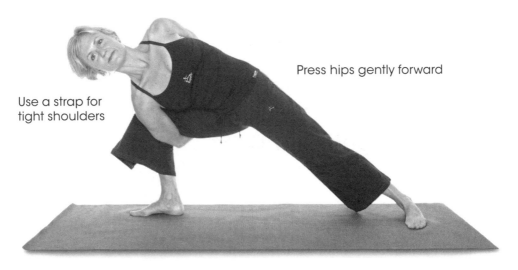

Use a strap for tight shoulders

Press hips gently forward

 A

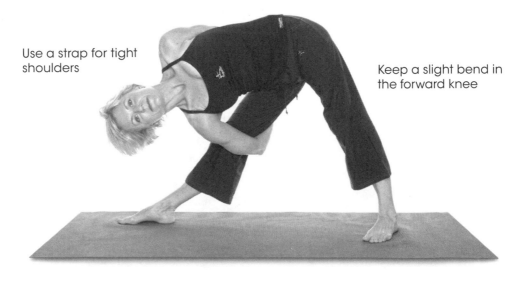

Use a strap for tight shoulders

Keep a slight bend in the forward knee

 B

Binding any yoga pose should allow for more freedom, not tie you in knots. Practice the Bound Triangle and Bound Angle poses within Mountain II for more heat, strength through your quads and waist, and openness through your chest and shoulders. Because you can no longer rely on your bottom arm to prop you up, support must come from within. Remember—as intensity increases, so does your need to breathe deeply.

Strengthens: Quads • Hip Flexors • Obliques
Stretches: Hip Adductors • Hamstrings • Chest • Shoulders

Getting into the pose

Bound Angle (A): From the Side Angle or Extended Angle pose, bring your forward hand inside your front foot. Reach behind your back with your top hand as you reach beneath your forward leg with your bottom hand, clasping them together. Lean back. Sink your hips toward the floor and roll your chest toward the sky.

Bound Triangle (B): From the Bound Angle, slowly straighten your forward leg, keeping a slight bend in your knee.

Holding the pose

Keep your back foot planted. Look up, down or forward, focusing on your breath. Switch sides.

Modification

If unable to clasp your hands, use a hand towel or strap. Begin by placing the strap in your top hand and reaching for it from below.

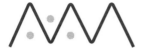

Chair and Balance Chair

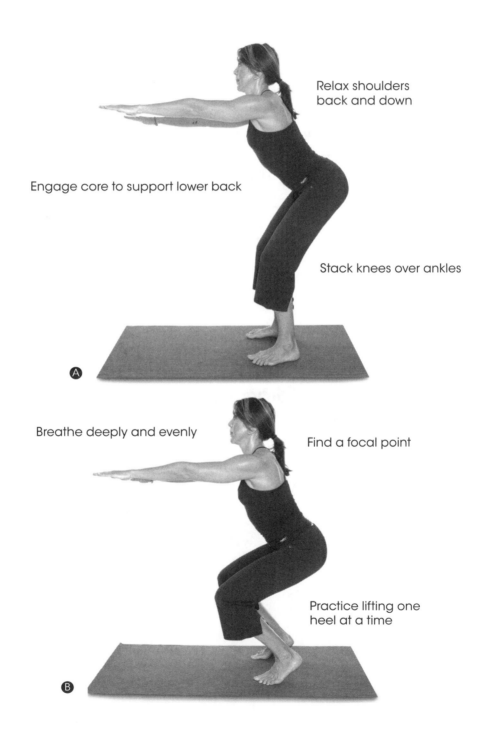

Relax shoulders back and down

Engage core to support lower back

Stack knees over ankles

A

Breathe deeply and evenly

Find a focal point

Practice lifting one heel at a time

B

In Mountain I, you move in and out of the Chair pose with every breath to warm up. In Mountain II, you hold the Chair or Balance Chair pose to increase stability, power, and strength in your lower body. The Chair pose is also included in Sun Salutations as part of Valley I.

Strengthens: Quads • Lower Back • Shoulders • Abdominals • Calves

Getting into the pose

Chair (A): Bend your knees and drop your buttocks, as if sitting in a chair.

Balance Chair (B): From the Chair pose, come up onto the balls of your feet and sit a bit lower. Keeping your chest lifted, find a focal point and breathe. Practice lifting just one heel at a time.

Holding the pose

Reach back with your tailbone. Lift your chest to the sky. Lift arms parallel to the floor, keeping elbows slightly bent. Support your low back by engaging your core. Keep your knees behind your toes by shifting your weight to your heels.

Modification

Rest hands on thighs for more support. For the Balance Chair, use caution if you're healing a foot or knee injury.

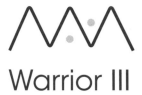

Warrior III

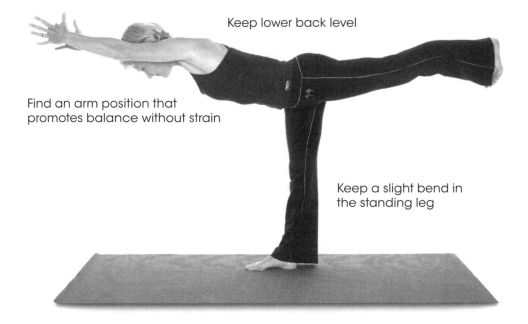

Keep lower back level

Find an arm position that
promotes balance without strain

Keep a slight bend in
the standing leg

Warrior III brings the strength and heat-building elements of a Warrior pose into the practice of balance (see p. 76 for the benefits of the Warrior poses). You can practice this dynamic pose within Mountain II or Valley II. If in Valley II, follow the pose with a second standing balance pose with your body upright to help regulate your blood pressure before coming to the floor for Mountain III.

Strengthens: Glutes • Upper Back • Lower Back • Abdominals • Concentration
Stretches: Hamstrings

Getting into the pose

Stand in the Mountain Pose (p. 66) with arms overhead or out to the side. Extend one leg back and hinge from your hips to lower your torso until both are parallel to the floor.

Holding the pose

Lengthen in opposite directions away from your navel. Breathe deeply to make your body longer and lighter. Switch sides.

Modifications

To decrease intensity, bring your arms out to the side or rest them lightly on the standing thigh. Bend or straighten your standing leg as needed for balance.

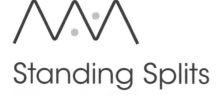

Standing Splits

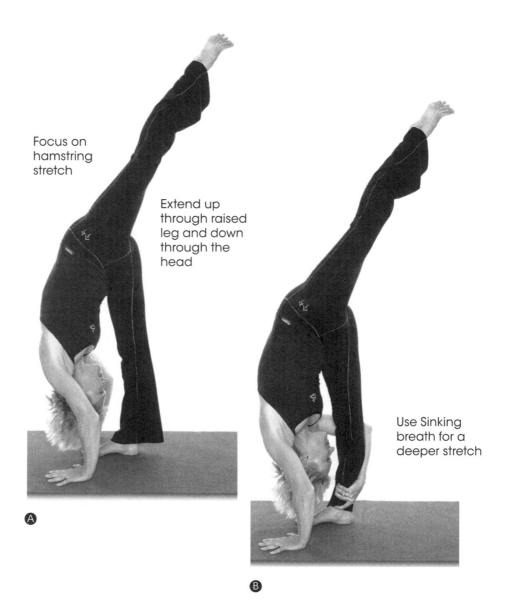

Focus on
hamstring
stretch

Extend up
through raised
leg and down
through the
head

Use Sinking
breath for a
deeper stretch

Ⓐ

Ⓑ

Like Warrior III, Standing Splits can be practiced within Mountain II or Valley II. If in Valley II, follow the pose with a second standing balance pose with your body upright to help regulate your blood pressure before coming to the floor for Mountain III.

Strengthens: Quads • Concentration
Stretches: Hamstrings • Hip Flexors

Getting into the pose

Place hands on the floor and lift one leg toward the sky while drawing your torso toward your thigh (A). For greater challenge, hold your standing ankle with one hand, keeping your other hand on the mat (B).

Holding the pose

Continue to reach up through your top leg and down through the crown of your head. Look at your big toe or back into your shin. Switch sides.

Modification

If you have tight hamstrings or trouble balancing, bend your standing leg as necessary.

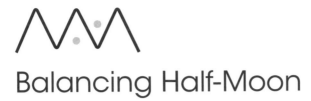

Balancing Half-Moon

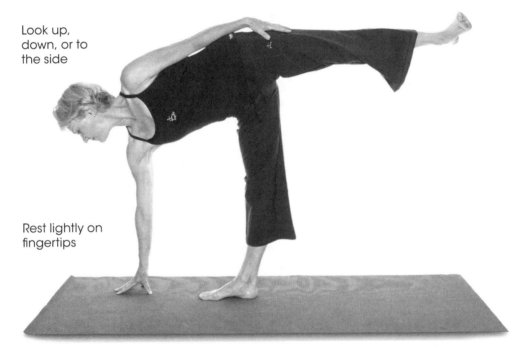

Roll chest toward sky

Look up, down, or to the side

Rest lightly on fingertips

You have the additional use of your hand in this balance pose, but you experience an added challenge of holding your spine parallel (or nearly parallel) to the floor. Practice this pose near the end of Mountain II or in Valley II when your body is *thoroughly* warm. In Valley II, follow this pose with an upright standing balance pose.

Strengthens: Obliques • Hip Abductors • Concentration
Stretches: Hamstrings

Getting into the pose

From the Standing Forward Fold pose (p. 106) or Pyramid pose (p. 114), raise your back leg level with your hip. Place your forward fingertips on the floor directly beneath your shoulder and your back hand on your hip. For a greater challenge, enter the Balancing Half-Moon from Warrior III or Standing Splits, bending your standing leg as necessary for balance and control as you transition.

Holding the pose

When balanced, roll your chest toward the sky and extend your top arm overhead. Then look up to your top hand. Stay focused, breathing deeply. Switch sides.

Modifications

If your hamstrings are tight, use a block. If you have shoulder instability or a rotator cuff injury, avoid this pose.

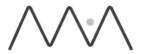

Tree

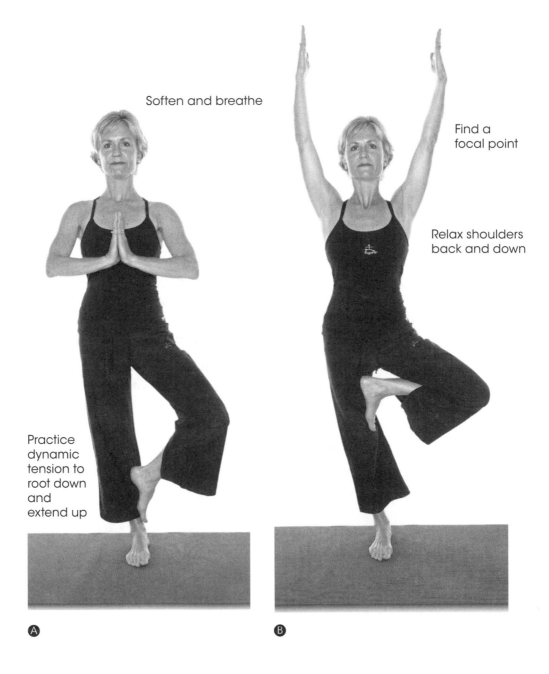

Soften and breathe

Find a
focal point

Relax shoulders
back and down

Practice
dynamic
tension to
root down
and
extend up

Ⓐ

Ⓑ

This popular Valley II pose promotes poise and calm. Visualize yourself as a tree, rooting down through your standing leg and expanding upward and outward like branches through your arms. Play with your arm and foot positions until you find a steady place to hold and breathe.

Strengthens: Hip Abductors • Abdominals • Shoulders • Concentration
Stretches: Latissimus Dorsi • Hip Adductors

Getting into the pose

Balance on one leg. Bring your opposite foot onto your standing ankle, calf, or inner thigh, avoiding the knee. Bring your hands into a prayer position (A). For a greater challenge, raise your arms overhead and look up (B).

Holding the pose

Lift up through the crown of your head while firmly rooting through your standing foot. Contract your abdominals and level your hips. Switch sides.

Modifications

If you have difficulty balancing, place the toes of your raised leg on the mat, or stand next to a wall for support. Use caution in this pose if you have knee concerns.

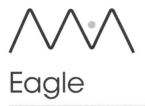

Eagle

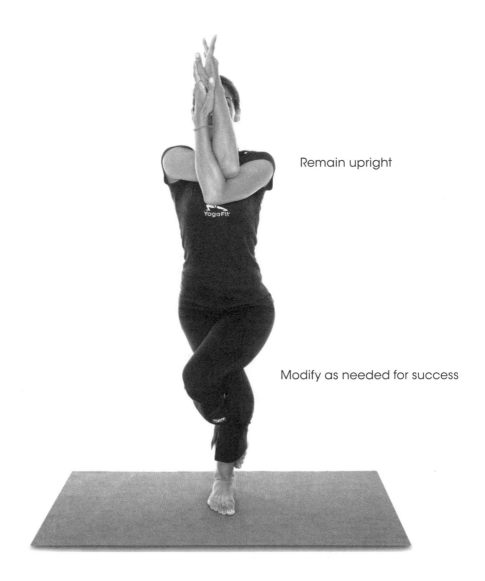

Remain upright

Modify as needed for success

Similar to the Tree pose, this Valley II pose works well after the body is warm to improve balance and focus.

Strengthens: Quads • Glutes • Hip Adductors • Concentration
Stretches: Glutes • Upper Back • Shoulders • Calves

Getting into the pose

Wrap your top leg around your standing leg. Touch your toes to the mat or hook your foot behind your calf. Sit back with your hips, keeping your spine upright. Wrap your arms to touch your palms (or back of your hands) together. The top leg is the same side as the bottom arm.

Holding the pose

Stretch upward and visualize drawing energy toward the sky as you root down through the standing foot. Contract your abdominals and keep your shoulders and tailbone low. Switch sides.

Modifications

If you feel unstable, stand near a wall for support. If you have knee concerns, use caution in this pose.

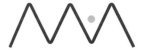

Standing Balance Pigeon

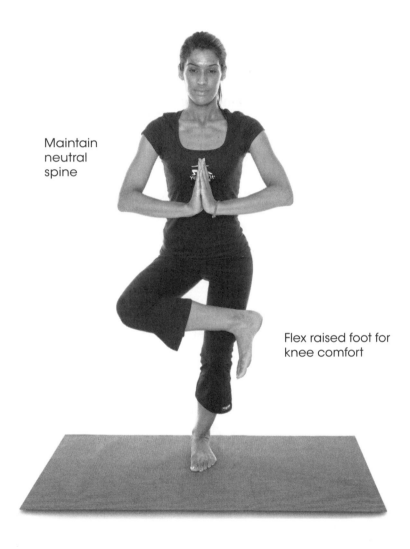

Maintain
neutral
spine

Flex raised foot for
knee comfort

In this Valley II pose, you gain all the benefits of balancing while getting a great hip stretch. This is a favorite of walkers, runners, and bikers. Because overworked, tense muscles respond well to heat, practice this pose when your body is thoroughly warm.

Strengthens: Quads • Lower Back • Concentration
Stretches: Hip Adductors • Hip Abductors

Getting into the pose

Begin in an easy Chair pose (p. 88). Shift weight to one foot. When balanced, place your opposite ankle across your standing thigh. Press through the heel of your lifted foot and bring your hands to your heart in a prayer position.

Holding the pose

Find a focal point and continue lengthening your spine with every breath. Engage your abdominals to support your lower back. Switch sides.

Modification

If you feel unstable, stand near a wall for support.

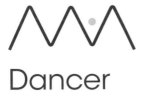

Dancer

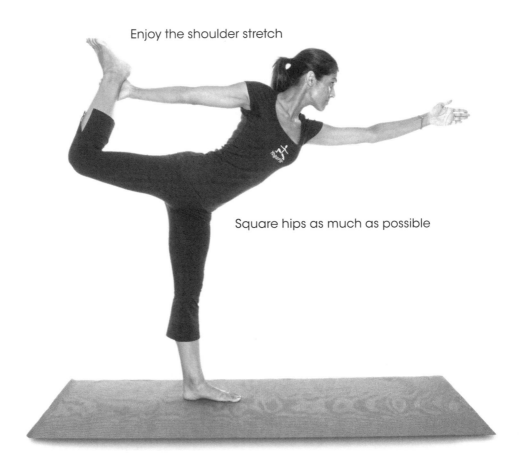

Enjoy the shoulder stretch

Square hips as much as possible

Do the Dancer pose in Valley II. Because this pose stretches the front of your hips and opens your chest, it relieves tightness caused by long periods of sitting, walking, running, or cycling.

Strengthens: Upper Back • Lower Back • Shoulders • Concentration
Stretches: Hip Flexors • Hamstrings • Quads • Shoulders

Getting into the pose

From the Mountain Pose (p. 66), balance on one foot. Bend your other leg and grasp the inside of your ankle with the hand on the same side, palm out. Reach your opposite arm to the sky and slowly hinge forward.

Holding the pose

Continue extending in opposite directions. Pull your ankle higher as you lift your forward arm. Square your hips with the front of mat. Switch sides.

Modification

If you feel unstable, place your hand on a wall in front of you for support.

7

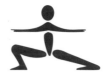

Forward and Backward Bends

Of all the yoga positions we practice, Westerners are perhaps most familiar with forward bending. Whether we're sitting at our desks, in our cars, at our dining room tables, or just reaching down to retrieve something from the floor, the forward bend is a position in which we spend much of our lives. So why practice it even more on our mats? Because most of our forward bending in daily life is done through our spinal column, where we round our shoulders and bend from the waist instead of hinging from the hips with a straight spine. Bending the way we do many times a day compromises our posture and leads to back pain and injuries. The more we practice hip hinging on our mats, the more likely we are to prevent back injuries off our mats.

As many hours as we spend bending forward, the opposite is true of bending backward. In fact, we don't spend nearly enough time in the backbend position. It's been said that our necks were created to allow us to look up at the stars, but how often do we really do this? In our forward-bending society we rarely extend our spines in any sort of backbend to perform daily tasks—and our habits are affecting our health. Studies indicate that slouching compresses our heart and lungs, maybe taking years off our lives. Poor posture can also lead to chronic pain and back injuries. Improving your posture does more than improve your physical health. We know that posture can reflect mood. The old saying "chin up!" suggests that sadness and defeat can cause us to slouch. Though the simple act of lifting your head and standing tall might not fix an unfortunate situation, it can certainly help you feel better. It's also known that back bending compresses your adrenal glands, located in your lower back, in a way that can energize you and prepare you for action.

> Forward bending and backward bending nourish your spine. Between each vertebrae of your spine are shock absorbers called disks. The only way to keep these disks soft and supple is by manipulating them through spinal movement. A YogaFit workout ensures that you move your entire spine in every direction—forward, backward, and sideways—through a range of motion that honors your body rather than injuring it.

Principles of Forward and Backward Bends

Several principles apply when practicing forward folds and backward bends.

- Breathe properly during forward and backward bends Breathing while holding poses helps to lengthen tight hamstrings and lower back muscles; it also relaxes you and fights the harmful effects of stress on your mind and body. Any time you're holding a forward bend, practice the Sinking breath technique (p. 23). Focus on completing your exhale and elongating and releasing muscles from the back of your legs, up your spine, to even that tight place between your ears. Any time you hold a backward bend, use the Expanding breath technique (p. 24), opening with every inhale, and holding the expansion with every exhale. Keep your head in line with your spine, allowing it to continue the curve either forward or back.

- Perform one of the two recommended warm-ups (described in chapter 10 beginning on page 200) for at least 15 minutes before practicing deep backbends.

- As you learned in SPA 1 (p. 6), when practicing backward bends, always begin with your base and work up. Also, be sure to engage your core to protect your back.

- Keep your knees slightly bent during all standing forward fold poses. If you have a lower back injury or a hamstring injury, bend your knees more to shorten the hamstrings for less strain on the muscles and decreased tension on the pelvis. When you allow your pelvis to tip forward into a folding pose you put less strain on your spine and the muscles of your lower back.

- Use counterposes to balance your body after deep stretches and releases, especially after vigorous backbends. Follow every backbend with a few breaths in a neutral spine position and then perform a forward bend. Or, if you're practicing backbends from the floor, such as the Bridge (p. 140) or Wheel pose (p. 142), follow with feet to the floor with knees bent, then knees to chest.

- The Swan Dive and Reverse Swan Dive are always used as the transition between the Standing Forward Fold pose and any upright standing pose (see Important Reminders in chapter 10, p. 202).

When it comes to our lower backs, all of us need to take care. When practicing backbends, most of us favor our lower backs. Although this method is easier, in the long run it can cause injury. The majority of Americans will at some point experience back pain. This is a shame because many of these injuries could be avoided through a program of strengthening and stretching that focuses on movement throughout the spine, not just the lower back, which is often the most flexible. When it comes to your spine in backward bends, focus on going long rather than deep—your back will thank you.

You'll perform forward bends and backward bends in Mountains I, II, and III (warm-up, workout, and cool-down). Milder backbends, such as the Cobra pose, are safe in Mountain I, but make sure your body is warm before you try the deeper backbends.

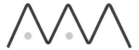

Standing Forward Fold

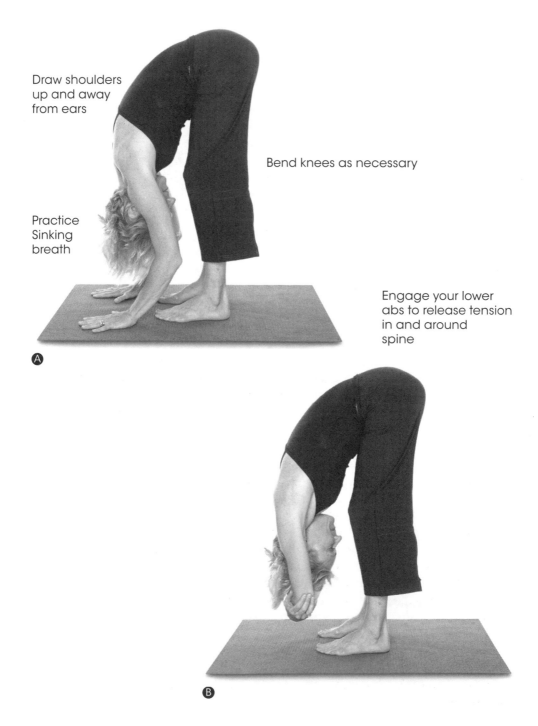

Draw shoulders up and away from ears

Bend knees as necessary

Practice Sinking breath

Engage your lower abs to release tension in and around spine

Ⓐ

Ⓑ

Use the Standing Forward Fold in Mountain I as a transition pose. Or use it in Mountain II as a place to hold and breathe, stretching your lower and middle back.

Strengthens: Quads • Hip Flexors • Abdominals
Stretches: Glutes • Hamstrings • Upper Back • Lower Back

Getting into the pose

Place your feet hip-width apart. Raise your arms overhead, bend your knees, and fold forward, leading with your chest. Extend your arms to the side as you bring your hands to the floor (A). For a greater challenge, if your lower back feels supported, grab your elbows and frame your face (B).

Holding the pose

Keep your knees bent to protect your lower back. Engage your abdominals as you lift your tailbone to the sky. Shake out your head and neck to release tension. Direct your breath into your back or hamstrings, wherever you feel the most tension.

Modification

If you have tight hamstrings or concerns about your lower back, place your hands on a block for support.

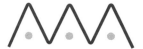

Downward-Facing Dog

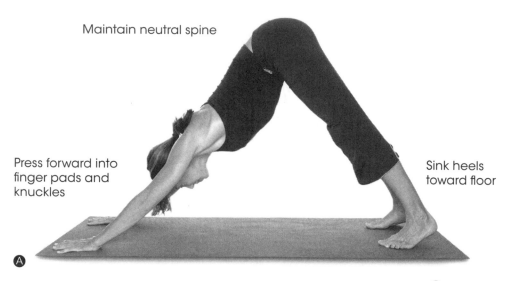

Maintain neutral spine

Press forward into
finger pads and
knuckles

Sink heels
toward floor

A

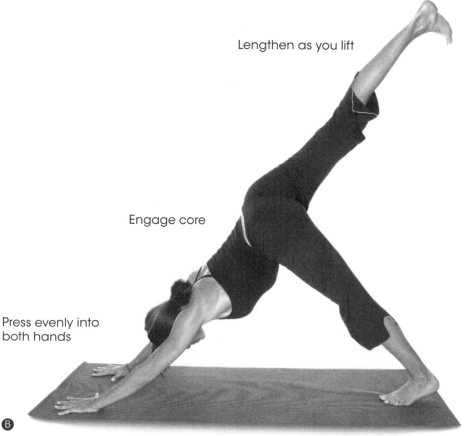

Lengthen as you lift

Engage core

Press evenly into
both hands

B

The Downward-Facing Dog (also called Down Dog), is the cornerstone of a flow yoga practice, as you saw in the Flow Series (p. 32) and will see again in the workouts in chapter 10. This pose is an excellent transition between other poses and provides strength and flexibility right where you need it. Use this pose often in Mountains I, II, and III.

Strengthens: Shoulders • Upper Back • Abdominals • Lower Back
Stretches: Glutes • Hamstrings • Shoulders • Calves

Getting into the pose

From the Child's Pose (p. 164), reach forward with your hands and press them into the mat with fingers spread wide. Lift your hips into an inverted V. Push back through the balls of your feet (A). For a greater challenge, lift one leg at a time to the sky (B).

Holding the pose

Keep your head between your arms as you lift your tailbone to the sky. Sink your heels toward the floor without rounding your back.

Modifications

If your back rounds, bend your knees. If you have shoulder or wrist concerns, remain in an extended Child's Pose (p. 164) or Dolphin pose (described next).

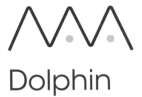

Dolphin

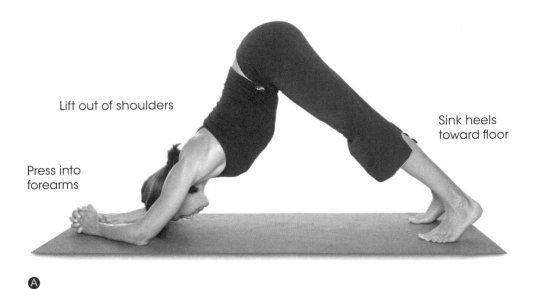

Lift out of shoulders

Press into
forearms

Sink heels
toward floor

A

Practice only if shoulders
are healthy and stable

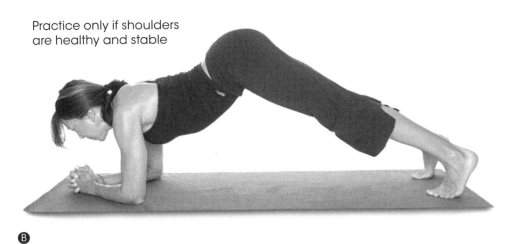

B

It's common to have imbalances in your upper body because you either favor one arm—athletes even more so—or neglect working your upper body altogether. The Dolphin pose is a great way to build strength and flexibility in and around your shoulders. Use this pose in Mountains II or III.

Strengthens: Upper Back • Shoulders
Stretches: Glutes • Hamstrings • Shoulders • Calves

Getting into the pose

Begin on your knees, with elbows above your shoulders. Interlace your fingers and press your forearms into the floor (A). Curl your toes and lift your hips. For the swimming Dolphin, inhale and draw your face over your hands (B). Then exhale and press back.

Holding the pose

Slowly straighten your legs as you sink your heels toward the floor. Look back at your toes and press the floor away with your arms. Lift your shoulders away from your ears.

Modification

If your back rounds, bend your knees.

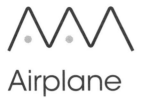

Airplane

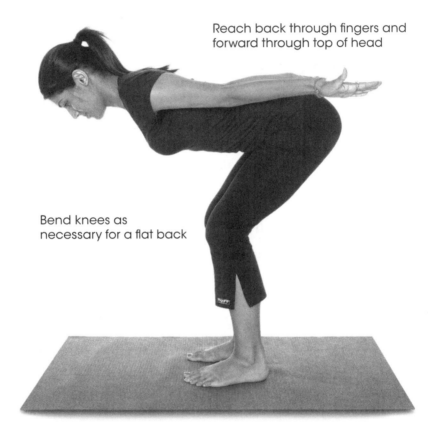

Reach back through fingers and forward through top of head

Bend knees as necessary for a flat back

The Airplane pose is ideal to use between forward bends and backward bends to elongate and stabilize the spine. Use it during Mountains I or II.

Strengthens: Quads • Lower Back • Abdominals
Stretches: Hamstrings

Getting into the pose

Standing, raise your arms overhead. Lower your arms to shoulder height and draw them back. With a slight bend in your knees, hinge forward halfway while maintaining a neutral spine (flat back). Draw your shoulder blades together and turn your palms toward the floor.

Holding the pose

Visualize pulling energy from your chest to your fingertips, keeping your back flat. Look down at the floor and reach forward through the top of your head. Lift your arms high to move your shoulder blades toward your spine.

Modifications

If you have lower back concerns, sciatica, or tight hamstrings, bend your knees deeply or place your hands on your thighs.

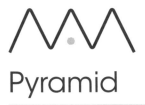

Pyramid

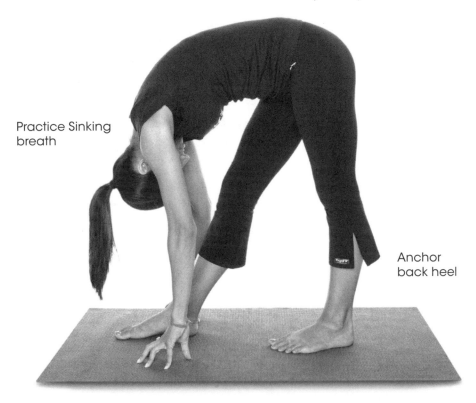

Square hips

Practice Sinking
breath

Anchor
back heel

Because your feet are in the same position here as for the Twisting Triangle (p. 148), the Pyramid often precedes or follows that pose in Mountain II. A longer exhale tells your nervous system it's time to relax; practice Sinking breath to help release tightness in your hamstrings.

Strengthens: Quads • Abdominals • Hip Abductors • Hip Adductors
Stretches: Glutes • Hamstrings

Getting into the pose

From a short Warrior I stance (p. 76), turn your back toes in until they nearly face the front of your mat. Square your hips and hinge forward over your front leg, reaching your forehead toward your knee.

Holding the pose

Keep your back heel anchored to the mat and soften your forward knee. Focus on the sensation in your hamstrings as you hold and breathe. Tighten your quadriceps for more strength and stability.

Modifications

To accommodate tight hamstrings, bend your front knee as necessary or place your hands on a block in front of your forward foot.

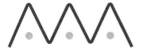

Standing Chest Expansion With Forward Fold

Engage abdominals

Draw shoulders
back and down

Bend knees as
necessary

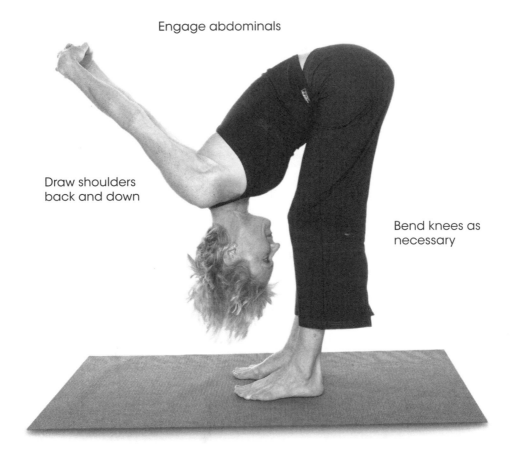

The chest muscles are some of the tightest muscles in the Western body. Studies show that poor posture, indicated by rounded shoulders and a slouched spine, can create heart problems. Spend a little time each day stretching your chest and breathing into an open heart and lungs. Use this pose before, during, and after any upper-body work to stretch shoulders and chest during Mountains I, II, or III.

Strengthens: Abdominals • Upper Back
Stretches: Hamstrings • Chest • Shoulders

Getting into the pose

From the Mountain Pose (p. 66), interlace your fingers behind your back and straighten your arms. Slowly raise your arms, bend your knees, and lower into a forward fold, leading with your chest.

Holding the pose

Breathe into your shoulders. Lift your tailbone to the sky and tighten your abdominals. Drop your head, but lift your shoulders away from your ears. Let every breath guide you deeper into the stretch.

Modifications

For lower back concerns, particularly disk injury or sciatica, remain standing with your knees slightly bent. If you're unable to clasp your fingers, use a strap or a hand towel.

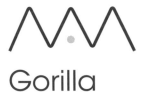

Gorilla

Focus on releasing lower back on exhale

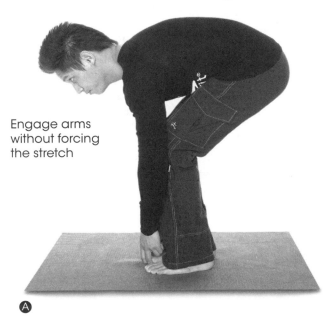

Engage arms
without forcing
the stretch

Ⓐ

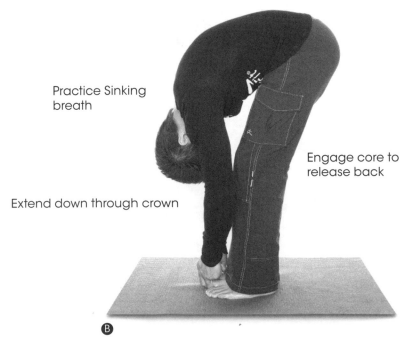

Practice Sinking
breath

Engage core to
release back

Extend down through crown

Ⓑ

These stretches are effective after Sun Salutations or following the Flow Series in Mountain II to offset the position of the wrists in Plank (p. 40), Crocodile (p. 42), and Upward-Facing Dog (p. 46).

Strengthens: Biceps
Stretches: Glutes • Hamstrings • Wrists

Getting into the pose

From the Standing Forward Fold (p. 106), grab your big toes with your index and middle fingers (A). Bring your elbows out to each side. Inhale and look up, straightening your spine. Exhale and draw the top of your head toward your feet. For a pose called the Wrist Stretch, from the Gorilla pose, flip your hands so that your palms face up. Slide your hands beneath your feet until your toes meet the inside of your wrists. Gently shift your weight forward toward your toes. Inhale and look up, straightening your spine. Exhale and draw the top of your head toward your feet.

Holding the pose

In both the Gorilla and the Wrist Stretch, slowly straighten your legs until you find a comfortable stretch (B).

Modifications

For lower back concerns, particularly disk injury or sciatica, place your hands on your thighs. Also place your hands on your thighs if you're unable to reach the floor. Remember to always bend your knees in forward folds.

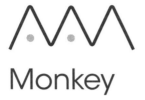

Monkey

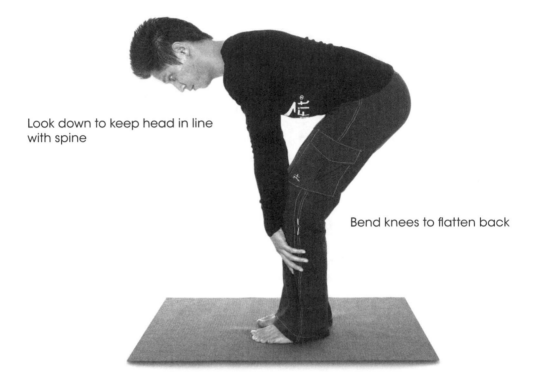

Look down to keep head in line with spine

Bend knees to flatten back

The Monkey pose is effective in Mountains I or II as a complement to forward bends. This pose activates the back, improving your posture and core strength.

Strengthens: Lower Back • Upper Back • Abdominals
Stretches: Glutes • Hamstrings

Getting into the pose

From the Standing Forward Fold (p. 106), place your fingertips on the floor in front of your feet. Inhale and lift your chest away from your thighs. Look up and straighten your back. Hold, or exhale back to the forward fold.

Holding the pose

Look slightly forward, keeping your back flat.

Modifications

For lower back concerns, particularly disc injury or sciatica, place your hands on your thighs. If you can't flatten your back with your fingertips on the floor, place your hands on your shins with your knees bent.

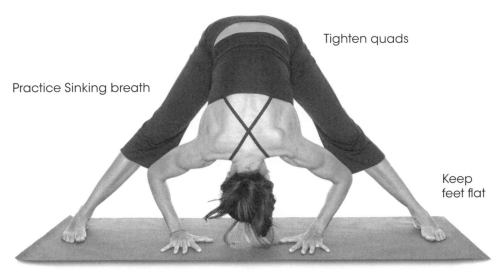

Standing Straddle Splits

Practice Sinking breath

Tighten quads

Keep feet flat

A

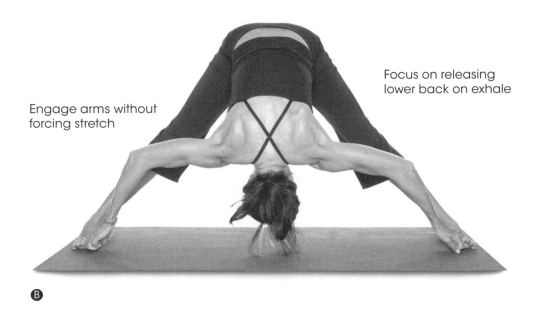

Engage arms without forcing stretch

Focus on releasing lower back on exhale

B

Use this pose in Mountain II, when your hamstrings are warm enough for a deep stretch.

Strengthens: Quad • Hip Flexors • Abdominals
Stretches: Hip Adductors • Hamstrings • Lower Back • Ankles

Getting into the pose

Stand with your feet apart and toes facing forward. Place your palms flat on the floor (if you can). Push your feet out, keeping the soles flat on the mat (A). For an added challenge, grab your big toes with your index and middle fingers (B), or interlace your fingers above your head for a chest expansion.

Holding the pose

Firm your quads while extending the crown of your head toward the floor.

Modification

If you have an ankle or groin injury, avoid this pose.

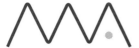

Seated Forward Fold

Practice Sinking breath

Use abdominals
to draw forward

Elevate
hips as
necessary

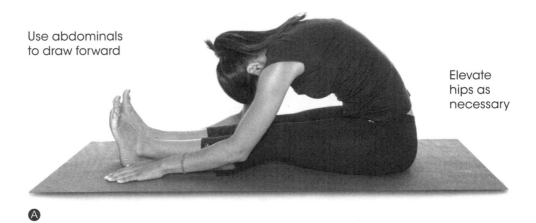

Ⓐ

Use abdominals to draw forward

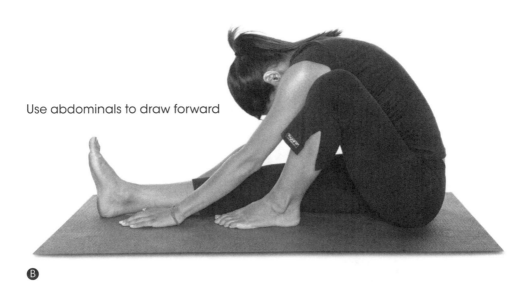

Ⓑ

This pose is used often in fitness as the benchmark for flexibility. As such, some people tend to become competitive, grab their feet, and pull themselves forward. This causes great harm to the lower back and does nothing to lengthen the muscles. Remember here the YogaFit Essence of listening to your body and letting go of expectations, judgments, and your competitive spirit. Draw forward from a desire to let go, not to win a competition. Use this pose in Mountain III, when your body is thoroughly warm.

Strengthens: Quads • Hip Flexors
Stretches: Glutes • Hamstrings • Lower Back

Getting into the pose

From a seated position, extend your legs. Pull your toes back toward your body. Reach forward, placing your hands on your legs, ankles, or feet, or on the floor. Draw forward through the top of your head using your abdominals (A). For an added challenge, bend one knee, bringing your foot flat to the floor with toes pointing forward. Keeping your knee pointing straight up, reach forward (B).

Holding the pose

Using a Sinking breath (p. 23), continue to reach forward toward your feet with your chest and the crown of your head. Firm your quads. Relax your shoulders back and down and enjoy the stretch.

Modifications

If you have tight hamstrings, sit on a folded blanket or rolled-up yoga mat, use a strap or hand towel around your feet, or bend your knees.

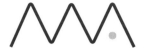

Seated Straddle Splits

Practice Sinking breath

Point toes straight up

Elevate hips as necessary

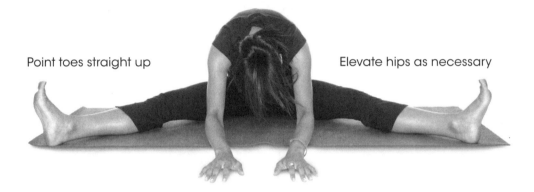

Use Seated Straddle Splits during Mountain III, after your body is thoroughly warm.

Strengthens: Quads • Hip Flexors
Stretches: Hip Adductors • Hamstrings • Lower Back

Getting into the pose

From a seated position, spread your legs wide. Hinge at your hips, place your hands on the floor in front of you, and use your abdominals to draw forward.

Holding the pose

Breathe into your back. Pull your toes back toward your body and point them toward the sky. Bend your knees as necessary.

Modifications

If you have tight hamstrings, sit on a folded blanket or rolled-up yoga mat, or bend your knees.

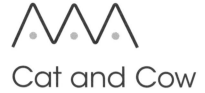

Cat and Cow

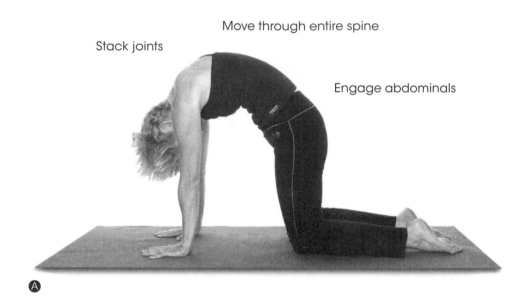

Stack joints

Move through entire spine

Engage abdominals

Ⓐ

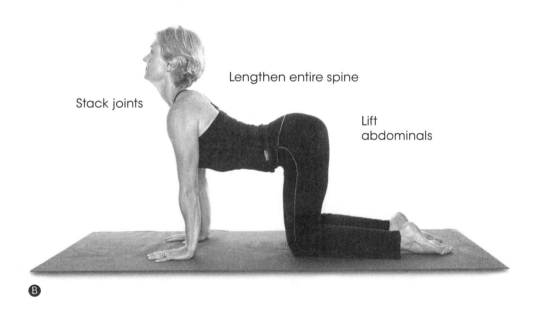

Lengthen entire spine

Stack joints

Lift abdominals

Ⓑ

Flow the Cat and Cow poses with your breathing to warm up your torso and spine in Mountain I. Or hold each pose individually in Mountains II or III.

Strengthens: Abdominals (Cat) • Upper Back (Cow) • Lower Back (Cow)
Stretches: Upper Back (Cat) • Lower Back (Cat) • Chest (Cow) • Abdominals (Cow)

Getting into the pose

Cat (A): From your hands and knees, with your shoulders over your wrists and hips over your knees, round your back to the sky.

Cow (B): From the Cat, arch your back and lift the chin.

Holding the pose

Keep your abdominals firm. In Mountain II, focus on lengthening through your entire spine, not just rounding (Cat) or arching (Cow) your lower back.

Modifications

If you have wrist discomfort or injuries, use "fists for wrists" with palms facing each other. For sensitive knees or other knee concerns, use a knee pad for comfort.

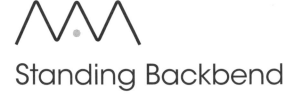

Standing Backbend

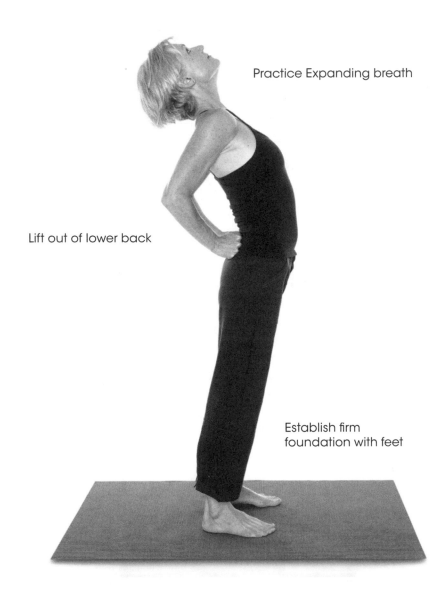

Practice Expanding breath

Lift out of lower back

Establish firm
foundation with feet

Improve flexibility in your spine by extending into a standing backbend. You'll feel the benefits immediately. Perform this pose near the end of Mountain II so that your body is very warm.

Strengthens: Glutes • Lower Back
Stretches: Chest • Shoulders • Hip Flexors • Abdominals

Getting into the pose

Moving slowly, firm your glutes and place your hands or fists on the bony points along your spine. Push your hips forward and lift your chest to the sky.

Holding the pose

Lift out of your lower back, drawing your elbows back to expand your chest. Look toward the sky without dropping your head back.

Modifications

If you have a lower back injury, do this pose with caution or use the Standing Chest Expansion With Forward Fold (p. 116) as an alternative. If your neck fatigues, look forward, tucking your chin slightly.

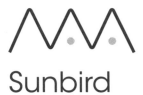

Sunbird

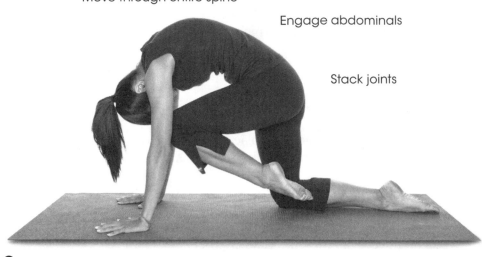

Move through entire spine

Engage abdominals

Stack joints

Ⓐ

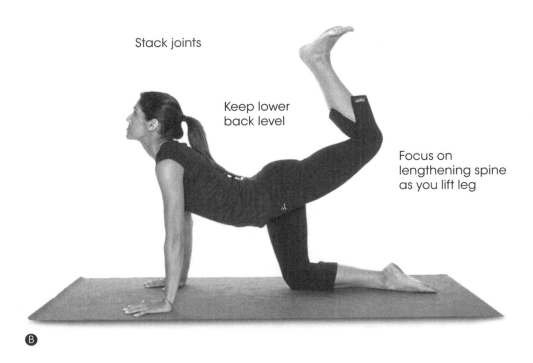

Stack joints

Keep lower back level

Focus on lengthening spine as you lift leg

Ⓑ

Like the Cat and Cow, do the Sunbird in Mountains II or III to build strength.

Strengthens: Glutes • Hamstrings • Lower Back • Arms
Stretches: Hip Flexors

Getting into the pose

From your hands and knees, exhale and bring one knee under your body toward your forehead (A). Then inhale and extend the same leg back and up toward the sky (B). Contract your abdominals throughout the movement.

Holding the pose

Move your energy from the center of your body outward. Keep the back of your neck long. Switch sides.

Modifications

If you have wrist discomfort or injuries, use "fists for wrists" with palms facing each other. For sensitive knees or other knee concerns, use knee pads for comfort.

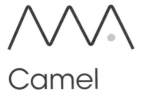

Camel

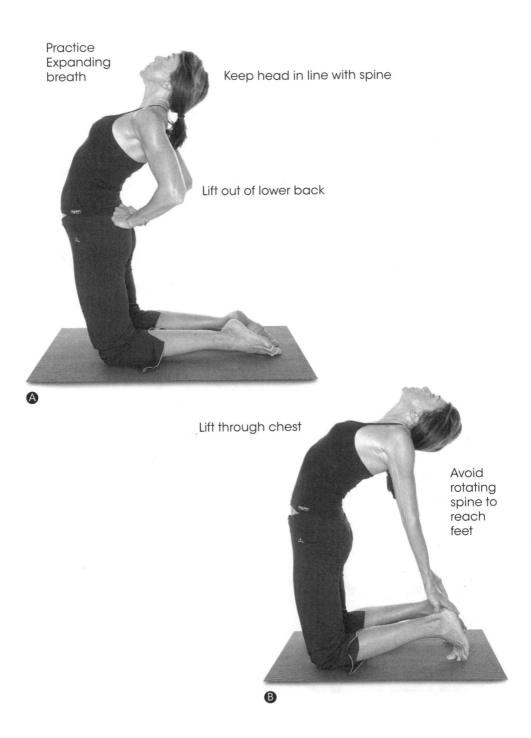

Practice
Expanding
breath

Keep head in line with spine

Lift out of lower back

Ⓐ

Lift through chest

Avoid
rotating
spine to
reach
feet

Ⓑ

Similar to the Standing Backbend, this pose works best when your body is warm. Because you're on your knees, use this pose in Mountain III.

> **Strengthens**: Glutes • Lower Back • Abdominals
> **Stretches**: Hip Flexors • Chest • Shoulders

Getting into the pose

Moving slowly from a kneeling position, place your hands or fists on the bony points along your spine. Firm your glutes, push your hips forward, and lift your chest toward the sky (A). For a greater challenge, drop your arms behind you and grab your heels (B).

Holding the pose

Lift out of your lower back, drawing your elbows back to expand your chest. Look toward the sky without dropping your head back.

Modifications

If you have a lower back injury, use caution with this pose or else, from a kneeling position, interlace your hands behind your back to stretch your chest in the modified version of Standing Chest Expansion With Forward Fold (p. 116). If your neck fatigues, look forward and tuck your chin slightly. For sensitive knees or other knee concerns, use a knee pad for comfort.

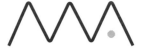

Locust and Superman

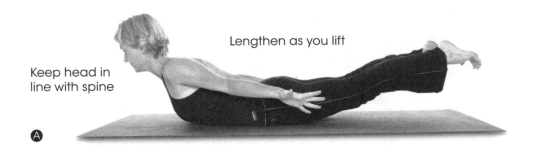

Keep head in
line with spine

Lengthen as you lift

Ⓐ

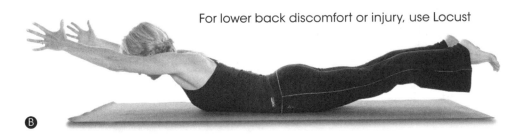

For lower back discomfort or injury, use Locust

Ⓑ

The Locust pose works well in Mountain III to safely stabilize and strengthen your lower back; it's a great pose to ward off back pain and injuries. The Superman offers the same benefits as the Locust when done in Mountain III but places more load on the lower back, so practice this pose only when your back is healthy and stable. Experiment with the Superman pose, picking the modification that builds strength without strain.

Strengthens: Glutes • Upper Back • Lower Back
Stretches: Hip Flexors • Abdominals • Chest

Getting into the pose

Locust (A): Lie on your belly with your arms at your sides, palms down. Engage your abdominals and glutes as you lift your upper and lower body off the ground.

Superman (B): Lie on your belly with your arms stretched above your head. Reach forward, engaging your abdominals and glutes as you lift your upper and lower body off the ground.

Holding the pose

In the Locust and Superman poses focus on lengthening more than lifting. Become longer with every breath. In the Locust, reach forward through the crown of your head and back through your toes; in the Superman, reach forward with your fingers and back through your toes.

Modifications

If you're a beginner or if you have a lower back injury, start these poses by folding your arms in front of your face and resting your forehead on your forearms in front of you. From this position, lift one leg at a time. Or lift just your upper body or just your lower body. As you develop strength and can hold these modifications for 5 to 10 breaths, try the Locust and then the Superman.

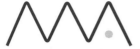

Bow and Half-Bow

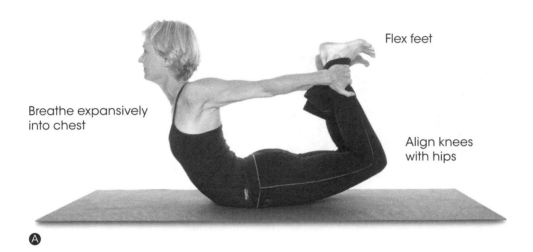

Breathe expansively into chest

Flex feet

Align knees with hips

A

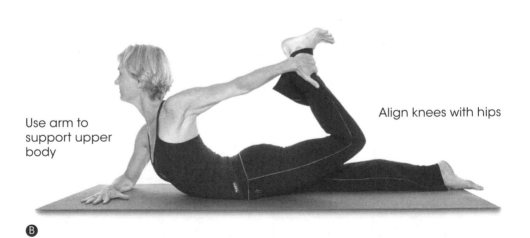

Use arm to support upper body

Align knees with hips

B

The Bow and Half-Bow poses create tension in order to release pent-up energy. Notice how relaxed and invigorated you feel after the effort of holding these poses for 5 to 10 breaths in Mountain III.

Strengthens: Quads • Glutes • Lower Back
Stretches: Hip Flexors • Abdominals • Chest • Shoulders

Getting into the pose

Bow (A): Lying on your belly, grab your right ankle with your right hand and your left ankle with your left hand. Lift your chest and legs to the sky. Pull your ankles back against your hands with your feet flexed, as if straightening your legs.

Half-Bow (B): Hold one ankle at a time, flexing your foot. Switch sides.

Holding the pose

Keep breathing into your chest as you open more with each inhale and lengthen out of your lower back.

Modification

If you can't reach your ankles, use a strap around your ankle.

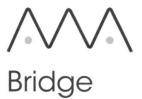

Bridge

Stack knees over ankles

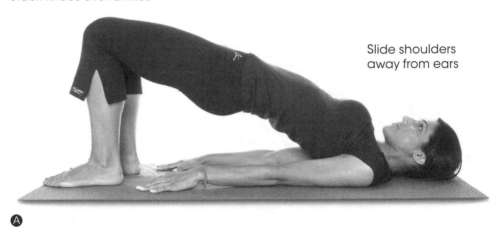

Slide shoulders
away from ears

A

Engage inner thighs
to keep knees stacked
over ankles

Keep your head still and centered

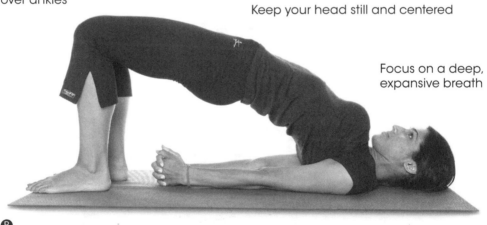

Focus on a deep,
expansive breath

B

The Bridge pose is an excellent way to stretch the front of your hips and open your chest, particularly if you sit for long periods or regularly walk, run, or cycle. This pose also targets muscles deep in your lower back and hips that are difficult to reach when upright. Move up and down with your breathing in Mountain I, or hold in Mountain III.

Strengthens: Glutes • Hamstrings • Hip Adductors • Lower Back
Stretches: Hip Flexors • Abdominals • Chest • Shoulders

Getting into the pose

Lie on your back with palms down. Slide your shoulders away from your ears. Bring the soles of your feet to the floor, hip-width apart. Press through your feet to lift your hips (A). For a greater challenge, interlace your fingers under your body. Walk your shoulders toward each other so your body is resting on the outside edges of your shoulders. Look toward your chest or the sky while focusing on your breath (B).

Holding the pose

Keep your head still to protect your neck (that is, don't look around). Use your inner thighs to keep your knees in line with your hips and toes. Breathe deeply into your open chest and navel.

Modification

Turn your palms up for more chest opening and core focus.

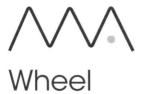

Wheel

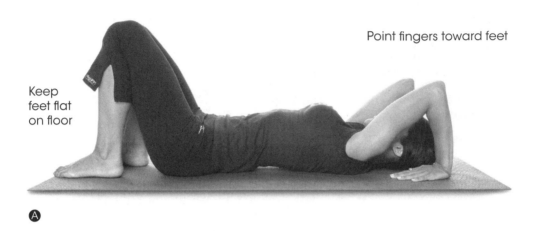

Keep
feet flat
on floor

Point fingers toward feet

A

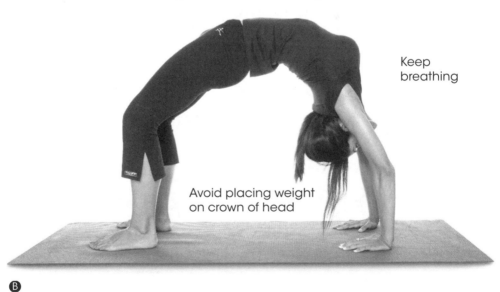

Straighten arms first, then legs

Keep
breathing

Avoid placing weight
on crown of head

B

Surprisingly, although you're in a backbend position, the Wheel is more of a shoulder opener than a backbend. Practice the Downward-Facing Dog (p. 108), the Dolphin (p. 110), or the Bridge (p. 140) to prepare for this energizing pose. Do this pose near the end of Mountain III when your body and mind are primed for a big stretch and a natural pick-me-up.

Strengthens: Glutes • Hamstrings • Lower Back • Upper Back • Shoulders
Stretches: Hip Flexors • Abdominals • Chest • Shoulders

Getting into the pose

After the Bridge pose, place both your hands on either side of your ears and point your fingers toward your feet. Place your feet flat on the floor hip-width apart (A). Press through your hands to lift your head and shoulders off the floor. Straighten your arms first, then your legs (B).

Holding the pose

Focus on stretching the front of your body without struggle or strain. To come out of the backbend, slowly place the back of your head on the mat as you return to the starting position. Bring your knees to your chest and relax.

Modifications

To build strength for the Wheel, keep your elbows bent and only come to the top of your head. Keep all your weight on your hands and feet (not your head and neck). Practice several push-ups, each one higher than the last. Come down slowly on the back of your head as you lower your back to your mat. Bring your knees to your chest and relax.

8

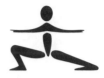

Twists

Your spinal work in YogaFit is not complete without twisting. Twists have a reputation for delivering instant gratification because their effects are felt almost immediately. Done properly, twisting poses target highly specialized muscles in the torso, building strength while releasing tension from deep within your body.

> Twisting poses likely affect more than just your spine. Yogis claim that through rotation you stimulate the organs of your abdomen and pelvis by wringing out old blood and excess fluid, allowing fresh blood and oxygen to flow in on release. Further, compressing and manipulating your intestines through twisting poses also improves digestion and elimination. The best way to know if these claims are true is to listen to your body—notice the changes that occur through your practice.

Before moving into any twisting pose, create space in your spine by practicing some of the SPA from chapter 1. Doing so should ensure the safest possible position for smooth and healthy movement. The SPA that pertain to twists are as follows:

- *Establish base and dynamic tension*. Like the stripe on a barbershop pole, twists begin at the lumbar spine and wind up the cervical spine. This upward spiral needs to be supported by a strong base. By anchoring your feet while drawing energy up through the arches of your feet and into the pelvic floor in standing poses like Twisting Triangle, and by keeping the base of your pelvis ("sit bones") anchored in seated twists, you support your pelvis. Through establishing a reliable foundation, rotation remains where you need it, in your spine.

- *Create core stability.* All twists should be initiated from a strong core—your waist and obliques—without leveraging with your arms too soon.
- *Align your spine.* Before moving into any rotation your spine must be in neutral position. This allows the vertebrae to rotate safely and smoothly on top of one another without pinching nerves or injuring the disks.
- *Relax shoulders back and down.* Drawing your shoulder blades down and back helps align your spine and engage your core.

> Always exercise attention and caution when practicing any form of rotation. Attend particularly to the position of your head and neck. It's common when rotating your head to also tilt it forward, backward, or to one side. Tilting can aggravate your neck, leading to tension or even injury. So, when twisting, you might try using mirrors to ensure that your head remains in line with your spine (SPA 3). Of course, if turning your head one direction is uncomfortable in a pose, look straight ahead, or even in the opposite direction. As long as you're in alignment and out of pain, your body will benefit.

In addition to the SPA, several other principles come into play when practicing twists.

- *Lead with your gut (belly) as opposed to your head (neck).* As mentioned, all twists begin at the base of the spine and slowly move up. The temptation in rotation is to set your sights on a deeper twist by turning your head first. However, because your neck is more flexible than the rest of your spine, your torso can't follow, and you're stuck with frustration. Rather than releasing tension, twisting in this way creates more tension. To make matters worse, you sometimes use an arm to pull yourself deeper into a twisting pose, rather than relaxing and allowing rotation to occur when your body is ready.
- *Engage root lock.* As described in chapter 3, before moving into any rotation, practice Mula Bhanda (root lock) to stabilize your lower back and pelvis.
- *Relax and let your breath be your guide.* With every inhale, continue to lengthen your backbone; with every exhale, soften into the spaciousness twisting allows. When you let go of forcing things and focus on the process, rather than on a final prize or goal, you gain much more.

All twists should be performed only when the body is thoroughly warm—so, within Mountains II or III.

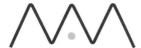

Twisting Lunge and Prayer Twisting Lunge

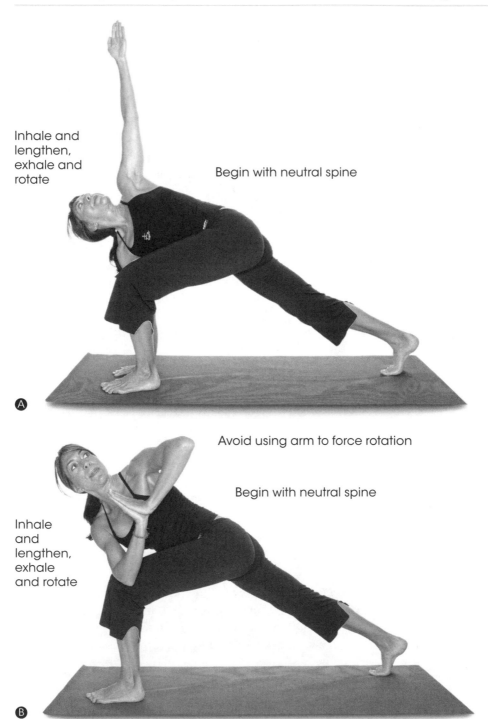

Inhale and lengthen, exhale and rotate

Begin with neutral spine

Ⓐ

Avoid using arm to force rotation

Begin with neutral spine

Inhale and lengthen, exhale and rotate

Ⓑ

Twisting Lunge and Prayer Twisting Lunge are practiced in Mountain II when your body is thoroughly warm.

Strengthens: Quads • Hip Adductors • Upper Back • Obliques
Stretches: Hip Flexors • Obliques

Getting into the pose

Twisting Lunge (A): From a lunge position with your left foot forward, place your right hand on the floor close to your left foot. With a straight spine, sweep your left arm up, reaching toward the sky.

Prayer Twisting Lunge (B): From a Kneeling Lunge, place your hands in prayer position over your heart. Rotate placing the back of your arm against the outside of your forward thigh. Lift your back knee off the mat and look upward.

Holding the pose

Press through your back heel and stack your forward knee over your ankle. Keep your chest close to your forward knee as you twist from the waist. Look up. Switch sides.

Modifications

For less intensity, drop your back knee to the mat for the Kneeling Lunge. Place your bottom hand on a block to lift your chest and bring your spine into neutral position for rotation.

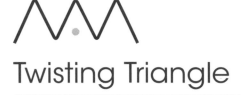

Twisting Triangle

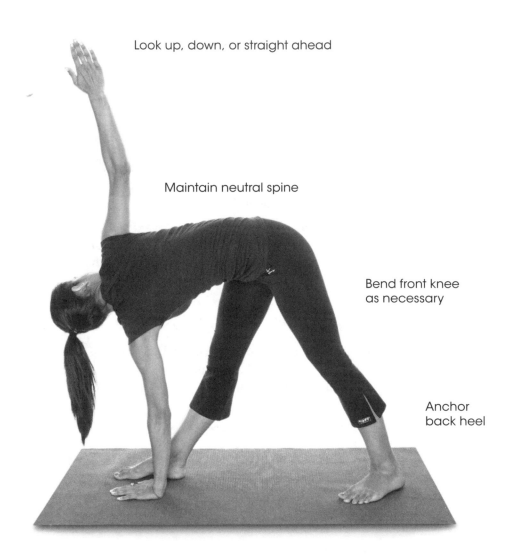

Look up, down, or straight ahead

Maintain neutral spine

Bend front knee
as necessary

Anchor
back heel

Twisting Triangle is a challenging pose that combines elements of forward folding, balancing, and twisting. Because the foot position is the same, Twisting Triangle typically follows the Pyramid pose (p. 114) in Mountain II.

Strengthens: Quads • Hip Adductors • Upper Back • Obliques • Shoulders
Stretches: Hamstrings • Lower Back • Upper Back • Obliques

Getting into the pose

From a short Warrior I stance, turn your back toes in until they nearly face the front of your mat. Square your hips and hinge forward over your front leg, keeping a slight bend in your front knee. If your right foot is forward, place your left hand on the floor to the right (or on your forward ankle). Twist to the right reaching your right arm to the sky.

Holding the pose

Keep your back heel anchored to the mat as you slowly straighten your legs. Lengthen your spine (rather than rounding forward) as you open your chest to the sky. Look up to your right hand. Switch sides.

Modifications

Bend your front knee or place your hand on a block to accommodate tight hamstrings. If you have a disk injury, use extra caution in this pose—the injury could be aggravated. Use the Pyramid pose as an alternative if necessary.

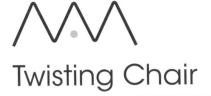

Twisting Chair

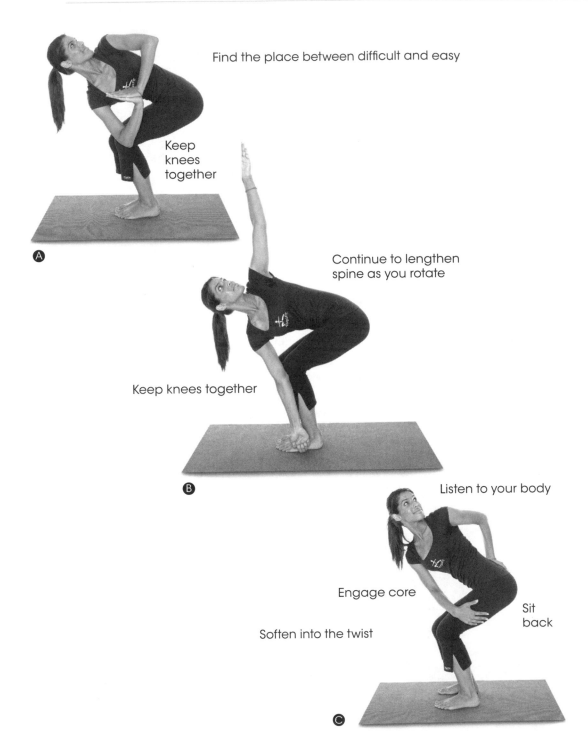

Find the place between difficult and easy

Keep
knees
together

A

Continue to lengthen
spine as you rotate

Keep knees together

B

Listen to your body

Engage core

Sit
back

Soften into the twist

C

This variation of the Chair pose (p. 88) is practiced only in Mountain II; it requires extra attention to alignment to prevent injuring your lower back.

Strengthens: Quads • Upper Back • Obliques
Stretches: Lower Back • Upper Back • Obliques

Getting into the pose

Start in the Chair pose with your feet and knees together. Lengthen your spine and place your hands in prayer position over your heart. Twist from the waist, placing your elbow on the outside of your opposite thigh (A). For an added challenge, place your bottom hand on the floor outside your foot. Reach up with your top arm as you roll your chest toward the sky (B).

When you're first learning this pose begin with a modified version in which you place one hand on your opposite thigh and the other on your lower back, focusing on keeping your knees together and your hips back (C).

Holding the pose

Engage your core to support your lower back. Inhale to lengthen. Exhale to twist. Keep your knees together as you release deeper into rotation.

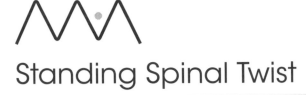

Standing Spinal Twist

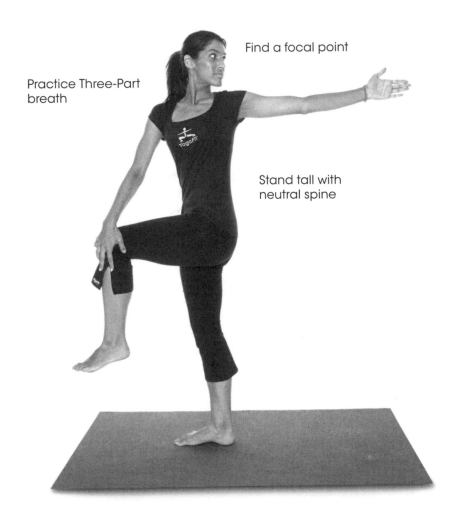

Practice Three-Part breath

Find a focal point

Stand tall with neutral spine

With the added element of rotation in a standing balance pose, you get twice the challenge and twice the benefit. Use this two-for-one pose in Valley II. Keep in mind that trying harder only makes the pose more difficult. Trade in willpower for a willingness to relax—trust in your body's innate ability to balance.

Strengthens: Upper Back • Obliques • Abdominals • Hip Flexors
Stretches: Hamstrings • Lower Back • Upper Back • Obliques • Shoulders

Getting into the pose

Standing tall in a Mountain Pose, lift your right leg. With your left hand, grasp your big toe with your index and middle fingers. Slowly press through your heel to straighten your leg and twist to the right.

Holding the pose

Place your right hand on your hip or open the arm behind you, following with your head. Keep your lower body strong; focus on your breath.

Modifications

As pictured, keep your knee bent (or use a strap) if you're unable to straighten your leg. Use a wall or chair behind you for more support.

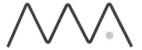

Seated Spinal Twist

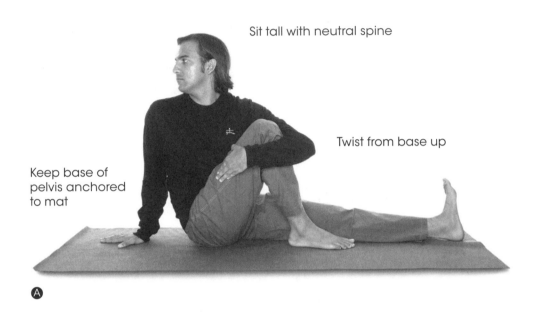

Sit tall with neutral spine

Twist from base up

Keep base of
pelvis anchored
to mat

A

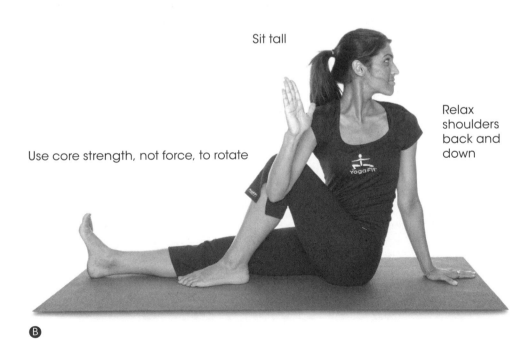

Sit tall

Relax
shoulders
back and
down

Use core strength, not force, to rotate

B

Do this pose in Mountain III to release your lower back while building strength in and around your spine.

> **Strengthens**: Upper Back • Obliques
> **Stretches**: Hamstrings • Lower Back • Upper Back • Obliques • Shoulders

Getting into the pose

From a seated position, extend your legs. Bring your right knee up with the sole of your foot on the floor. Place your right hand next to you or behind you and sit tall. Beginning at the base of the spine, rotate to the right, bringing your left forearm around to hold your right shin (A). Use your core strength rather than your arm to deepen the twist. For an added challenge, place your left elbow outside your right knee (B). Hold and breathe.

Holding the pose

Use only your core strength to deepen the twist. Lengthen your spine with every inhale; twist further with every exhale. Switch sides.

Modification

If you have difficulty keeping your back straight, sit on a rolled-up yoga mat or folded blanket. Elevating your hips relieves tension caused by tight hamstrings that can tip the pelvis back, making it difficult to sit with a neutral spine.

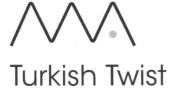

Turkish Twist

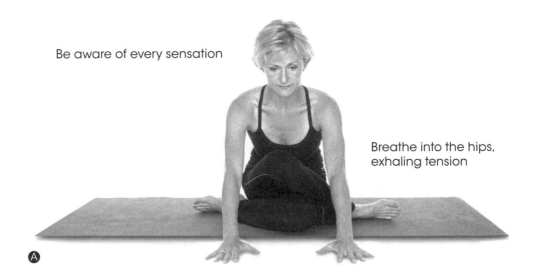

Be aware of every sensation

Breathe into the hips, exhaling tension

A

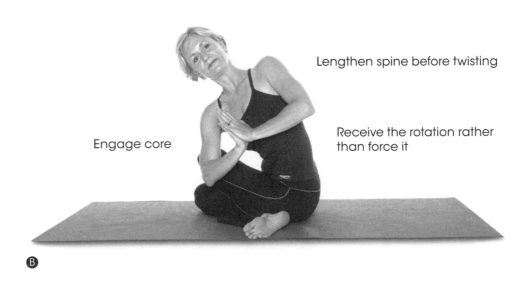

Lengthen spine before twisting

Engage core

Receive the rotation rather than force it

B

This Mountain III pose offers all the benefits of rotation combined with a deep hip stretch.

Strengthens: Upper Back • Obliques
Stretches: Hip Abductors • Glutes • Lower Back • Upper Back • Obliques

Getting into the pose

Cross one knee over the other. Draw your feet back toward your hips. First, sit tall and relax into the hip stretch by drawing your forehead toward your knee on the exhale (A). Use the Sinking breath technique (chapter 3) to help release tension. Then sit tall and place your hands in prayer position over your heart. Rotate toward your top leg, placing your elbow on your thigh (B).

Holding the pose

Inhale to lengthen. Exhale to rotate. Hold for 5 to 10 breaths. Switch sides.

Modifications

If one hip lifts off the floor, sit on a rolled-up yoga mat or folded blanket. If you have knee pain or difficultly stacking your knees, do the Seated Spinal Twist instead.

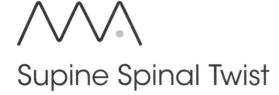

Supine Spinal Twist

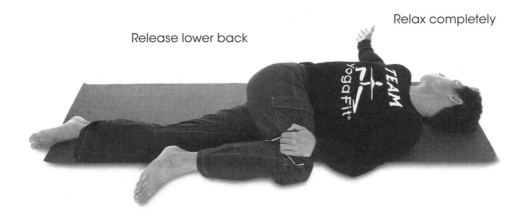

Release lower back

Relax completely

Use this pose to release your lower back after standing postures. The pose works well near the end of Mountain III to prepare your body for the Final Relaxation pose.

Stretches: Hip Abductors • Lower Back • Upper Back • Obliques

Getting into the pose

Lie down on the floor. From the Knees to Chest pose (p. 182), extend your left leg along the floor. Place your right foot on the floor and push to lift, and shift your hips slightly to the right. Use your left hand to gently draw your right knee toward the floor.

Holding the pose

Keeping both shoulders on the floor, look to the right. Practice Sinking breath for optimal release and relaxation. Switch sides.

Modifications

If you have a disk injury, the rotation and flexion in this pose might aggravate the injury. In this case, place both feet on the floor and lower your legs together to one side.

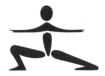

9

Deep Relaxing Stretches and Inversions

At the end of a YogaFit workout, or following any physical exercise, your body is warm and your muscles fatigued. This is the optimal time to practice deep relaxing stretches and inversions. When you turn up your internal thermostat in Mountains I and II, your muscles and connective tissue become more pliable and can lengthen effectively without injury. When you're wrung out, physically and mentally, your mind and body are more willing to relax and release muscular tension caused by strength training (Mountain II) or stress.

Deep Relaxing Stretches

As we've mentioned, deep relaxing stretches are best done in Mountain III, the cool-down segment of your YogaFit workout. The stretches we'll look at in this chapter are these:

- Child's Pose
- Kneeling Lunge and Crescent Lunge
- Quad Stretch
- Kneeling Shoulder Stretch
- Revolving Knee to Head
- Frog
- Butterfly

- Upside-Down Pigeon
- Supine Half-Lotus
- Knees to Chest
- Dead Bug
- Big Toe Hold
- Fish
- Final Relaxation

These stretches, or poses, are designed to increase flexibility in your muscles and joints and to release stress and tension. Note that the Seated Forward Fold and Seated Straddle Splits from chapter 7 (pp. 124 and 126) are also considered deep relaxing stretches to be incorporated into Mountain III.

Two of the primary benefits of deep relaxing stretches are to maintain functional flexibility and release stress.

- *Maintaining functional flexibility.* Yoga poses are known for requiring exceptional flexibility, but as far as your health is concerned it's far more important to maintain functional flexibility—the ability for your body to move easily through a normal range of motion. Your body's level of functional flexibility is compromised by everything from sports training to the natural aging process. Without regular stretching, your muscles atrophy (shrink), you lose your ability to take a deep breath, and your joints become stiff or even immobile.

- *Relaxation and stress release.* Holding deep stretches creates relaxation and releases stress. Even mental stress builds muscular tension, which must eventually be released if you are to enjoy good physical health. As you hold these poses, monitor your body for tightness and rigidity. Breathe deeply into tense areas and, as you exhale, consciously work to dissolve the tension. This is mind–body work that you should do daily.

> For a muscle to lengthen and maintain its new shape, it must be held in a stretch for at least 30 to 45 seconds. Thus, you should hold every Mountain III pose for 5 to 10 breaths, slowing down each inhale and exhale so your body has time to relax and elongate. Just as you must exercise regularly to maintain strength and reduce stress, you must stretch often to maintain flexibility. That's why yoga is a practice meant to be enjoyed for a lifetime.

Inversions

Inversions are done at the end of Mountain III, your cool-down phase. The three inversions we'll look at are:

- Legs Up Wall
- Plow
- Shoulderstand

In addition to the health benefits already mentioned for the deep stretches, some inversions also increase strength and flexibility, whereas others are extremely relaxing. All inversions prepare your mind and body to "let go" during the Final Relaxation pose.

The health benefits of being upside down are many. The medical community has begun to realize what yoga practitioners have taught for thousands of years: Inversions have a positive impact on your mental and physical well-being. There are several benefits of turning upside down:

- You reverse the pull of gravity, allowing venous blood to flow easily back to your heart and lungs for improved circulation.
- You improve blood flow to your brain for a natural pick-me-up and improved concentration.

- You relieve varicose veins and spider veins.
- You reduce your heart rate and blood pressure.
- You boost your immune system.
- You create traction in your spine, removing pressure from the disks between your vertebrae.

> Studies show that chronic stress increases your risk of obesity, depression, heart disease, and much more due to elevated levels of a hormone called cortisol. Though cortisol is useful in circumstances that require immediate energy and action, too much can be harmful. Yoga can lower your cortisol levels. Deep breathing, deep relaxing stretches, and a focused mind all help to calm the "fight or flight" response and induce a healing state of relaxation.

Note that two of the three inversions we'll look at, the Plow (p. 190) and Shoulderstand (p. 192), are not recommended for certain conditions, including pregnancy, high blood pressure, glaucoma and other eye conditions, neck injury, or cervical arthritis. Ask your doctor which inversions are appropriate for you. In Mountains I, II, or III, rest and check in with your body in the Child's Pose.

Heat and Flexibility

Most people think of stretching as a way to increase flexibility and reduce injury. Flexibility is usually defined as the ability to move a joint through its full range of motion (ROM). As a technique to reduce injury, many assume that stretching before exercise or athletic activity helps prepare muscles for movement. However, research cannot confirm that flexibility exercises done before elevation of core body temperature are effective in reducing injury.

Two essential properties of muscles allow them to stretch: elasticity and plasticity. The elastic properties of muscles allow them to return to their original state after a stretch. If they didn't, the muscles would lengthen continuously until they became so loose that no movement was possible. The plastic properties of muscles allow them to adapt to the continued stress placed on them, and to retain those adaptations. If muscles were not plastic, you wouldn't be able to strengthen or stretch them; they would remain the same. Interestingly, both of these qualities, elasticity and plasticity, become more evident when there's an elevation in core body temperature. Another way of saying this is that muscles improve more rapidly if you work them when they are warm.

Thus, once you have sufficiently elevated your core body temperature, you can begin using movements that condition your body for greater strength, stretch, and flexibility. Your deepest flexibility stretches will occur near the end of your workout, when your body is warmest and your muscles' elasticity and plasticity are optimal.

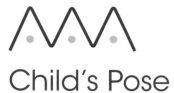

Child's Pose

Use this pose to rest and check in with your body

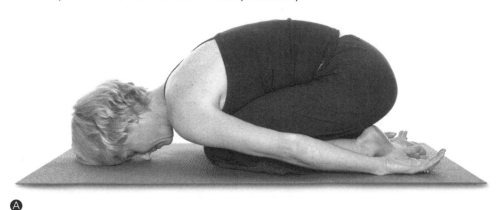

Ⓐ

Draw shoulders back and down

Rest or transition
into next pose

Spread fingers wide

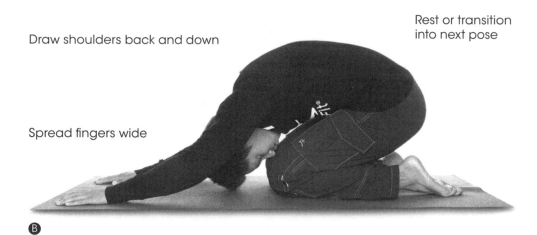

Ⓑ

Child's Pose is a Mountain I, II, and III pose. To ensure this is a comfortable position for you to rest and reflect, try both variations of this pose, the wide-knee Child's Pose and the extended Child's Pose.

> **Strengthens**: Mind–Body Connection
> **Stretches**: Lower Back • Glutes • Shoulders (extended Child's Pose)

Getting into the pose

Begin kneeling on all fours. Push back and bring your arms around to the sides of your body (A). To stretch your shoulders or to transition to another pose, reach your arms out in front of you for an extended Child's Pose (B). To make more room for your body, separate your thighs for a wide-knee version of the Child's Pose.

Holding the pose

Rest and breathe, allowing your body to completely relax.

Modifications

Rest your head on your fists or your chest on a block for greater back and neck support. If you have knee pain or discomfort, place a rolled-up yoga mat or folded blanket behind your knees.

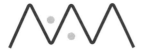

Kneeling Lunge and Crescent Lunge

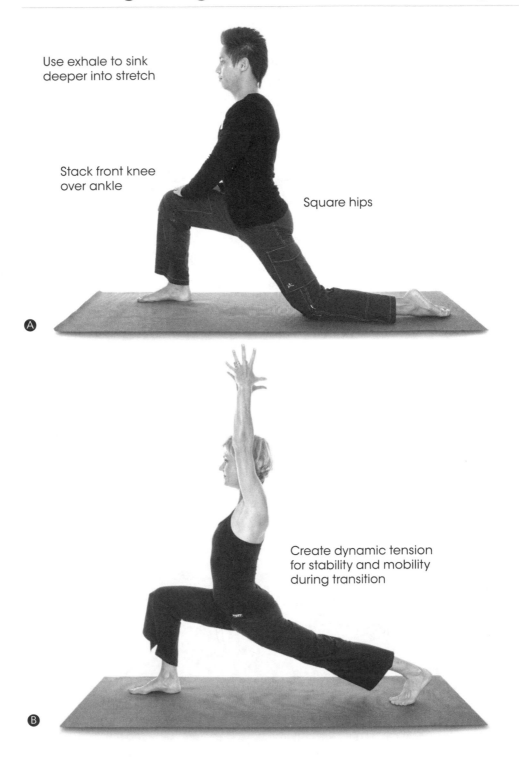

Use exhale to sink deeper into stretch

Stack front knee over ankle

Square hips

Ⓐ

Create dynamic tension for stability and mobility during transition

Ⓑ

The Kneeling Lunge and Crescent Lunge open the front of your hips, which tend to tighten after long periods of sitting, running, or cycling. Stretching your hip flexors helps keep you standing upright, preventing lower back problems. Do the Kneeling Lunge and Crescent Lunge during Valley I as part of Sun Salutations and within your Mountain II work.

Strengthens: Quads • Hamstrings
Stretches: Hip Flexors • Quads

Getting into the pose

Kneeling Lunge (A): From all fours, place one foot forward between your hands, stacking your knee over your ankle.

Crescent Lunge (B): Lift your back knee off the floor and straighten your back leg, pressing your back heel toward the wall behind you.

Holding the pose

In either pose, face forward and place your hands on your forward thigh or at your heart in prayer position, or raise your arms overhead. Sink through your hips. Switch sides.

Modification

In the Kneeling Lunge or Crescent Lunge, reduce the intensity by placing your fingertips on the floor.

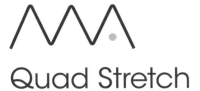

Quad Stretch

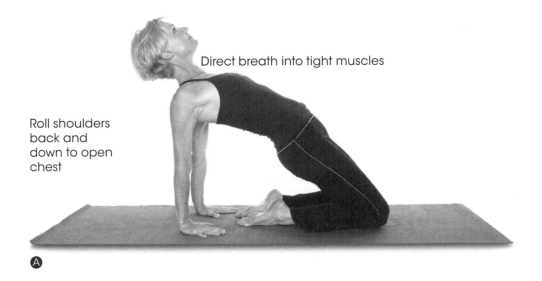

Roll shoulders
back and
down to open
chest

Direct breath into tight muscles

Ⓐ

Explore feeling maximum sensation without pain

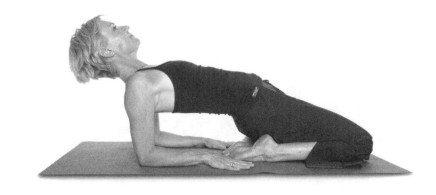

Ⓑ

Although we rely on our quadriceps daily for strength and power, most of us tend to stretch them far less than we do their counterpart, the hamstrings. Use this pose in Mountain III to release and lengthen these workhorse muscles.

Strengthens: Glutes
Stretches: Quads • Hip Flexors • Chest • Shoulders

Getting into the pose

From a kneeling position, sit back on your heels. Place your hands on the floor next to your hips. Lift your hips and chest to the sky (A). For a greater challenge and a deeper stretch, place your forearms on the floor (B).

Holding the pose

In both versions of the pose, increase the stretch by pushing your hips forward and lifting your chest.

Modifications

If you have a knee injury or discomfort, or tight quadriceps, place a chair, step, or bench behind you for support.

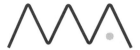

Kneeling Shoulder Stretch

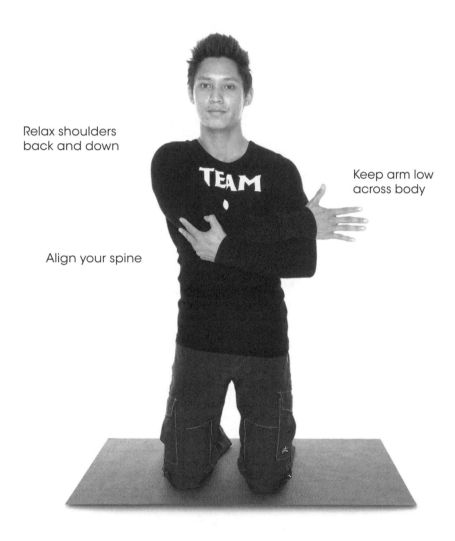

Relax shoulders
back and down

Keep arm low
across body

Align your spine

This pose is helpful for swimmers, weightlifters, and other athletes with tight upper backs and shoulders. Practice it near the beginning of Mountain III before you come down onto your back.

Stretches: Shoulders

Getting into the pose

From a kneeling position, draw one arm low across the front of your body. With your opposite hand, hold your triceps and gently stretch the back of your shoulder.

Holding the pose

Sit up tall as you continue gently drawing your arm low across your body.

Modification

If you have a knee injury or discomfort, practice this pose in an upright seated position.

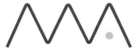

Revolving Knee to Head

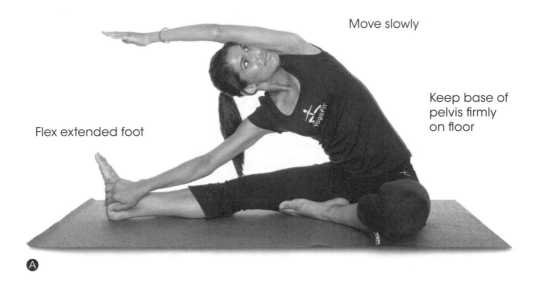

Move slowly

Keep base of
pelvis firmly
on floor

Flex extended foot

Ⓐ

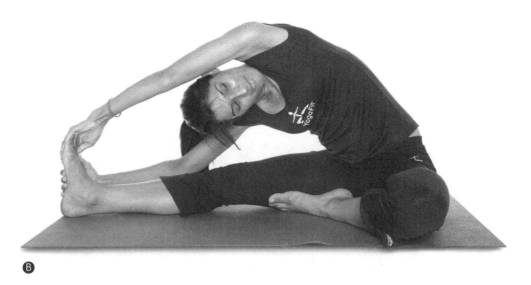

Relax, rather than pull, into the stretch

Ⓑ

This Mountain III pose is a deep stretch for the upper and lower body and also strengthens your torso. Come out of this pose slowly and with awareness to protect your back.

Strengthens: Quads • Lower Back • Obliques
Stretches: Hamstrings • Hip Adductors • Chest • Shoulders • Obliques

Getting into the pose

From Seated Straddle Splits (p. 126), bend one knee, placing the sole of your foot on your inner thigh. Keeping both sit bones (the bony points at the base of the pelvis) on the floor, slide your bottom hand down the inside of your leg toward your foot. Reach your top arm over your head, coming into a side bend. Place your bottom hand on your extended leg, or grab the outside edge of your extended foot. Roll your chest as you reach your top arm to the sky (A). For a greater challenge, lower your top arm over your ear, reaching for your extended foot (B).

Holding the pose

Continue opening your chest while drawing your shoulder blades down your back. Firm your quads to help release your hamstrings. Switch sides.

Modifications

If you have a knee injury or discomfort, keep both legs extended in Seated Straddle Splits (p. 126). If you're unable to reach your extended foot with your bottom hand, use a strap.

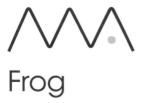

Frog

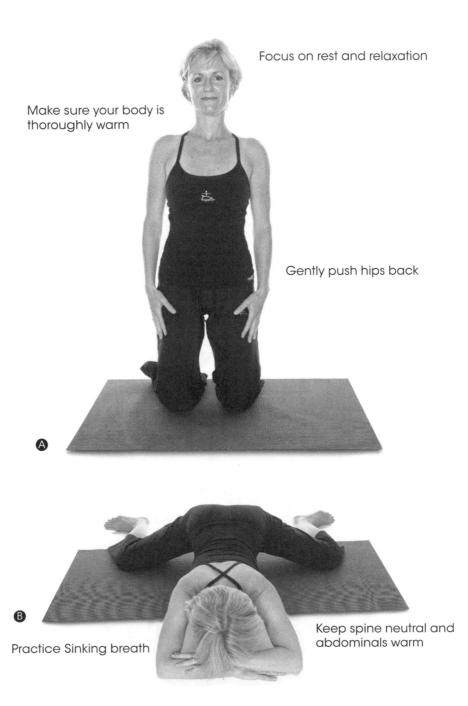

Focus on rest and relaxation

Make sure your body is thoroughly warm

Gently push hips back

Ⓐ

Ⓑ

Practice Sinking breath

Keep spine neutral and abdominals warm

Try the Frog pose in Mountain III to stretch tight inner thigh muscles after the demanding strength work you do for your legs in Mountain II. Succumb to gravity in this pose for total body relaxation.

Stretches: Hip Adductors

Getting into the pose

Begin kneeling, facing the long edge of your mat (A). Separate your knees out wide to each side, keeping your ankles directly behind your knees and your feet flexed. Slowly lower your upper body toward the floor (B).

Holding the pose

Gently push your hips back, keeping your spine neutral and abdominals firm. Use the Sinking breath technique (p. 23) to help release muscular tension.

Modifications

For knee injuries or discomfort, use a wide-knee Child's Pose (p. 164) or a Dead Bug pose (p. 184).

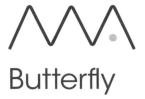

Butterfly

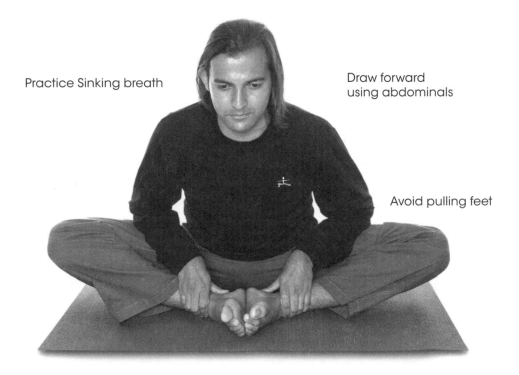

Practice Sinking breath

Draw forward
using abdominals

Avoid pulling feet

Use the Butterfly after your body is warm, during Mountain III. This pose is a favorite among athletes with tight hips and inner thighs, such as bikers and runners, as well as individuals who sit for long periods.

Strengthens: Abdominals • Hip Flexors
Stretches: Hip Adductors • Glutes • Lower Back

Getting into the pose

Sitting tall with a straight spine, place the soles of your feet together in front of you. Use your outer thighs to draw your knees toward the floor. Holding your ankles, use your abdominals to fold forward.

Holding the pose

Keeping your elbows back along your body, continue to draw your knees toward the floor. Use Sinking breath (p. 23) to help release muscle tension.

Modification

If you are unable to maintain a straight spine, sit on a rolled-up yoga mat or folded blanket.

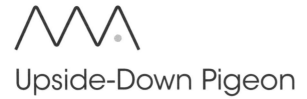

Upside-Down Pigeon

Flex both feet

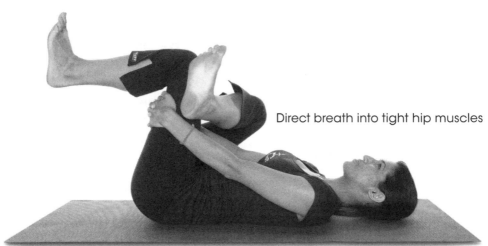

Direct breath into tight hip muscles

The Upside-Down Pigeon is a deep stretch that releases your hips, where you store much of your tension and stress. Releasing this area allows you to experience more agility and balance in your body and mind. Because you do this pose on your back, completely supported by gravity, it also restores and relaxes your spine. Use this pose near the end of Mountain III, before you begin inversions.

Stretches: Hip Adductors • Hip Abductors • Glutes

Getting into the pose

From your back, lift your right foot off the floor and place your left ankle across your right thigh, flexing both feet. Hold your right hamstring with both hands and gently draw your right knee toward your chest until you feel a stretch in your left hip.

Holding the pose

With each exhale, continue drawing your knee close, focusing on releasing your left hip. Switch sides.

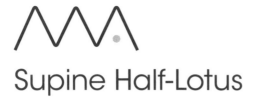

Supine Half-Lotus

Move slowly and listen to your body

Relax completely

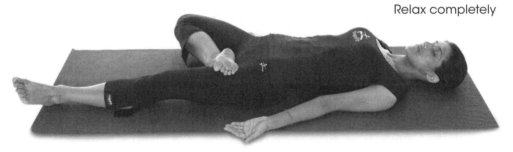

Because you're on your back, the Supine Half-Lotus allows your entire body to relax. For this reason, it's particularly beneficial near the end of Mountain III.

> **Stretches**: Hip Adductors

Getting into the pose

From your back, place one foot on your opposite thigh near the top of your leg. Allow the knee of your bent leg to relax toward the floor. Proceed carefully and with great awareness, without forcing your knee into the pose.

Holding the pose

Monitor your body for any sign of tension or resistance. With every exhale, release this tension. Switch sides.

Modification

If you have knee pain or discomfort, do the Upside-Down Pigeon instead.

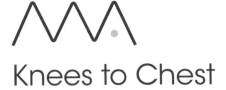

Knees to Chest

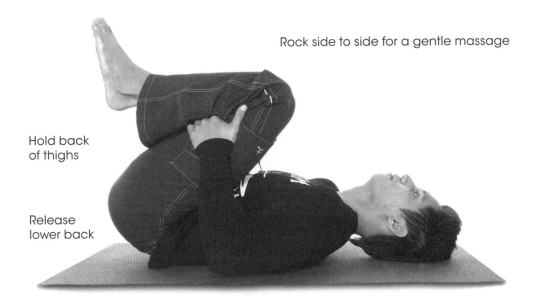

Rock side to side for a gentle massage

Hold back
of thighs

Release
lower back

Similar to the Child's Pose, Knees to Chest is a restorative, restful place to return to any time during Mountain III that you need a break. Also use this pose following backbends to release your lower back and neutralize your spine.

▶ **Stretches**: Glutes • Lower Back

Getting into the pose

Lie down with your back on the floor. Bring your knees into your chest. Hold onto the back of your thighs.

Holding the pose

Keep drawing your knees toward your chest while keeping your tailbone on the floor. For a gentle back massage, rock side to side.

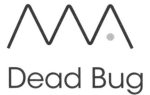

Dead Bug

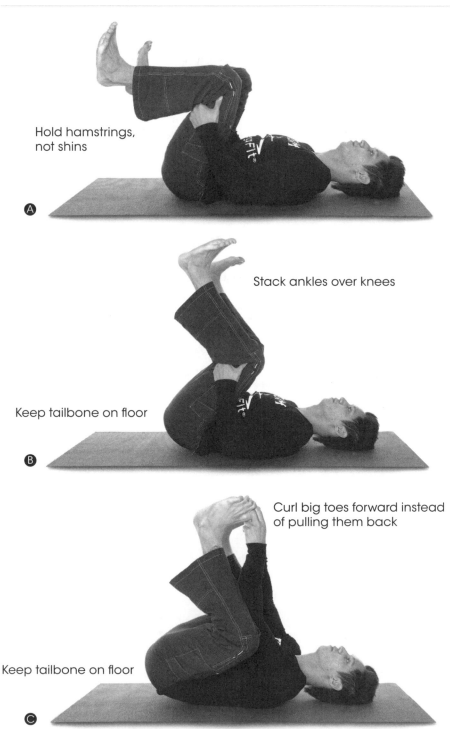

Hold hamstrings, not shins

A

Stack ankles over knees

Keep tailbone on floor

B

Curl big toes forward instead of pulling them back

Keep tailbone on floor

C

Practice this pose near the end of Mountain III, before you begin inversions.

Strengthens: Biceps
Stretches: Hip Adductors • Glutes

Getting into the pose

From the Knees to Chest pose, hold your hamstrings and draw your knees down toward the floor (A). When your tailbone is resting on the floor, lift the soles of your feet toward the sky (B). For a greater challenge, grab your big toes with your index and middle fingers and draw your knees toward the floor while bringing your elbows out to each side. Keep your ankles stacked over your knees (C).

Holding the pose

In all versions of this pose, continue drawing your knees toward the floor. Rest your head, shoulders, and tailbone on the floor as you stretch. Allow yourself to feel supported here by gravity as you release physical and emotional tension from your back and hips.

Modifications

If this pose is uncomfortable, stay in the Knees to Chest pose. If your tailbone lifts off the floor, keep your knees bent, as shown in photo A.

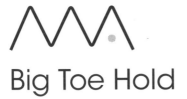

Big Toe Hold

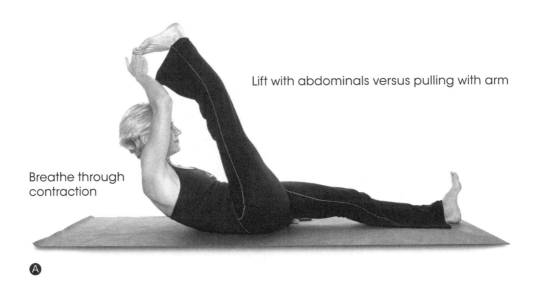

Lift with abdominals versus pulling with arm

Breathe through
contraction

Ⓐ

Anchor opposite hip to floor

Relax and breathe deeply

Ⓑ

This two-for-one pose strengthens your abdominals while increasing flexibility in your legs. Use this pose in Mountain III.

Strengthens: Abdominals • Hip Flexors
Stretches: Glutes • Hip Adductors • Hamstrings

Getting into the pose

From your back, lift your right leg. Grab your big toe with the index and middle fingers of your right hand and place your left hand on your left thigh. Exhale, lifting your forehead toward your knee and hold for five breaths (A). Inhale, releasing your head back to the floor as you open your leg to the same side. Look over your opposite shoulder and hold for five breaths (B). Inhale, again lifting your leg back to center and your forehead toward your knee; hold for five breaths. Release and switch sides.

Holding the pose

When your leg is extended to the side, keep both hips on the floor. Press through your heels and straighten your legs.

Modifications

If you have tight hamstrings, use a strap across the ball of your foot, or keep your knee bent throughout each phase of the pose.

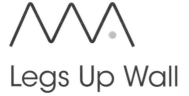

Legs Up Wall

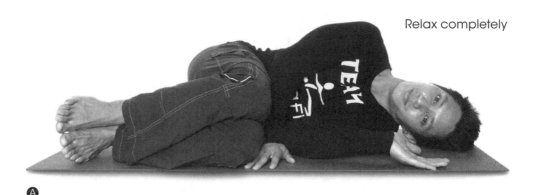

Relax completely

Ⓐ

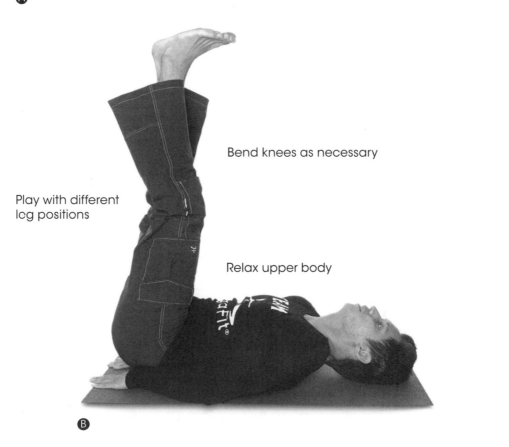

Bend knees as necessary

Play with different leg positions

Relax upper body

Ⓑ

In this Mountain III inversion, it's hard not to relax. To add a deep, relaxing stretch, experiment with different leg positions, such as straddle splits or a pose similar to the Butterfly (p. 176), in which the soles of your feet are together and your knees are open. Remember to check with your doctor before doing any inversions.

Stretches: Glutes • Hamstrings • Hip Adductors (if legs apart)

Getting into the pose

From the Knees to Chest pose, roll over onto one side until your glutes touch the wall (A). Use your hands to roll onto your back, straightening your legs up the wall (B).

Holding the pose

Separate your legs slightly to breathe more easily into the bottom of your lungs.

Modification

Without a wall available, make fists and place them under your hips for support.

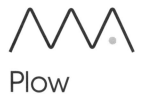

Plow

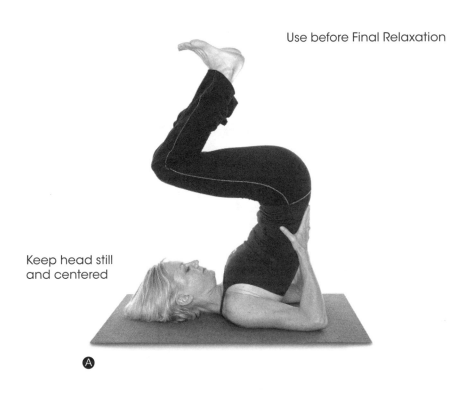

Use before Final Relaxation

Keep head still
and centered

Ⓐ

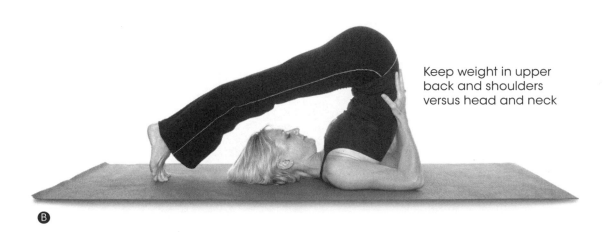

Keep weight in upper
back and shoulders
versus head and neck

Ⓑ

The Plow is most effective in Mountain III near the end of your session, when your body is thoroughly warm. Because the Plow compresses the throat, it's believed to stimulate the thyroid gland, increasing metabolism. Remember to ask your doctor which inversions are appropriate for you.

Strengthens: Abdominals
Stretches: Glutes • Lower Back • Hamstrings

Getting into the pose

Lying on your back, use your abdominals to bring your legs over your head (A). Support your low back with your hands as you slowly straighten your legs and place your toes on the floor (B).

Holding the pose

Keep your legs straight. If your feet don't touch the floor, support your lower back with your hands. Breathe into your throat.

Modifications

As we mentioned at the start of the chapter, the Plow is not recommended for people with certain medical conditions. As an alternative, and with your doctor's permission, practice the Legs Up Wall pose instead. If your toes don't reach the floor in Plow, place the tops of your feet on a chair.

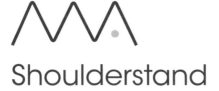

Shoulderstand

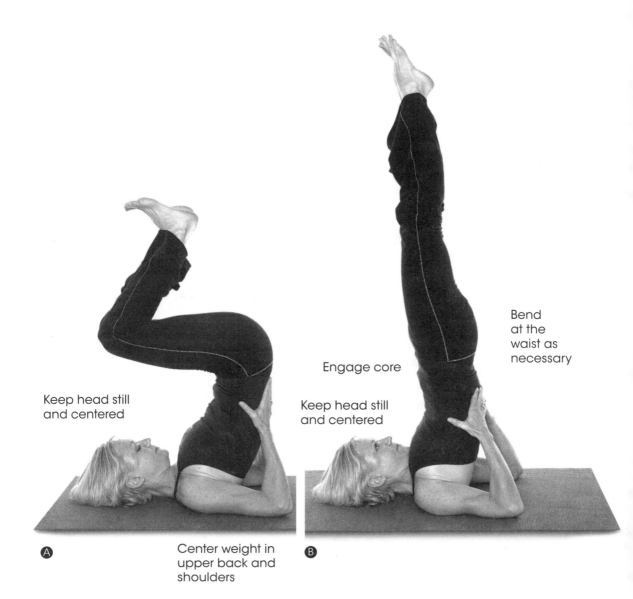

Keep head still
and centered

Center weight in
upper back and
shoulders

Ⓐ

Engage core

Keep head still
and centered

Bend
at the
waist as
necessary

Ⓑ

The Shoulderstand is an inversion that follows the Plow pose at the end of Mountain III. Like the Plow, this pose is believed to stimulate the thyroid gland, increasing your metabolism. Again, remember to ask your doctor which inversions are appropriate for you before you try them.

Strengthens: Upper Back • Abdominals • Lower Back • Glutes
Stretches: Shoulders • Chest

Getting into the pose

From the Plow, bend your knees and support your back with your hands as you lift your legs to the sky (A). Don't move your head or neck. For an added challenge, straighten your legs and continue lifting them to the sky until your body is perpendicular to the floor (B). For less pressure on your neck, keep a slight bend at the waist; again, don't move your head or neck.

Holding the pose

Keep a slight bend at the waist and knees for less pressure on your neck. Breathe into your throat. Always follow with Knees to Chest.

Modifications

As we've mentioned, like the Plow pose, the Shoulderstand is not recommended for people with certain medical conditions. As an alternative, and with your doctor's permission, practice the Legs Up Wall pose instead.

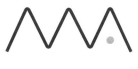

Fish

Check in with your body

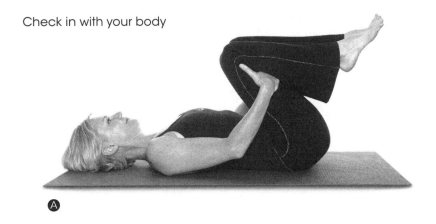

(A)

Practice Expanding breath

Open throat without dropping head back

Bring legs together

Point toes

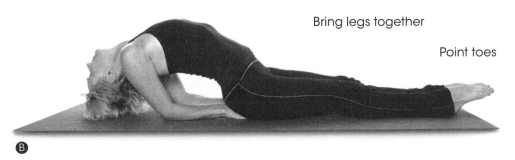

(B)

The Fish pose is an effective counterpose when practiced directly after the Plow and Shoulderstand at the end of Mountain III. This pose can alleviate certain chest disorders and promote a healthy heart. The pose might also stimulate the thyroid, increasing metabolism.

Strengthens: Upper Back
Stretches: Chest • Throat • Shoulders

Getting into the pose

From the Plow or Shoulderstand, bring your knees to your chest (A). Extend your legs along the floor and slide your hands under your hips, palms down. Bring your elbows toward each other beneath your back (B). Point your toes toward the floor as you reach back in the opposite direction with the crown of your head, shifting your body back slightly as well.

Holding the pose

Lift your chest and rest your head lightly on the floor, maintaining space in the back of your neck; relax. Your breath should feel deep and easy; if it doesn't, adjust your position. Always follow with Knees to Chest.

Modification

As necessary, place a rolled-up yoga mat or folded blanket under your upper back for support.

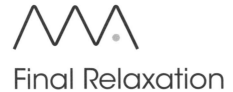

Final Relaxation

Stay present in the moment
Breathe naturally
Relax completely

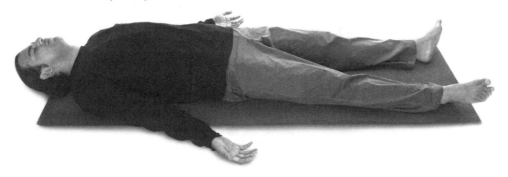

At the end of a YogaFit session you have completed your work out and prepared your mind and body for your work in. Many yoga teachers remind us that you should never confuse activity with productivity, and this is particularly true in the Final Relaxation pose. This is the one pose in which you are instructed to do nothing, and yet you receive a lot.

The Final Relaxation pose allows you an opportunity to again become aware of your body and mind, mentally and physically integrating the benefits of your practice. It also provides an important transition back into your daily routine. Finally, this pose helps release muscular tension and stress for improved health and well-being.

The Final Relaxation pose is an integral part of any yoga practice and should never be rushed or skipped. At the end of Mountain III, allow at least 6 to 10 minutes for Final Relaxation.

Relaxes: Everything!

Getting into the pose

Lie on your back, or in any position that allows you total comfort and relaxation. Turn your palms toward the sky and allow your feet to roll open.

Holding the pose

Let your breath return to its natural, rhythmical cycle. Continue to release stress and tension, finding peace and calm.

Modifications

For lower back discomfort, place your feet flat on the floor and bend your knees, allowing them to lean against one another. For added comfort, place a pillow or towel behind your knees or your head.

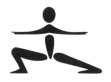

Part III

Putting It All Together

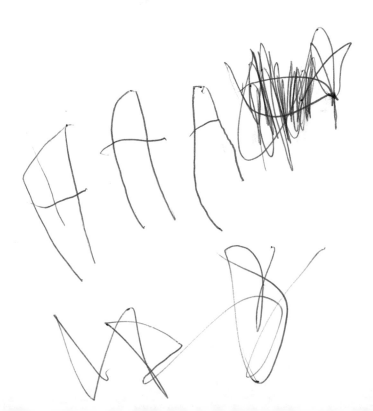

10

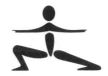

Workouts for Fitness and Sports

It's time now to begin your personal YogaFit practice by selecting and following a YogaFit workout that matches your level of expertise and physical condition. In our workouts you'll work all your body parts, including your legs, arms, torso, sides, shoulders, neck, back, abdominals, and inner organs. Each workout combines standing poses with seated and lying-down poses, and progresses from a warm-up with heat-building sequences to deep, relaxing stretches and a cool-down. Each pose in each workout is followed by an appropriate counterpose (e.g., a backbend is followed by a forward bend) to keep your body tuned and balanced.

Sometimes you might need to modify or omit poses that are not recommended or appropriate for you because of a medical condition, or if they feel uncomfortable. Be cautious with special conditions, such as injuries or pregnancy; before you begin a workout, review Special Considerations for YogaFit (p. 10) in chapter 1. Also remember to consult your doctor before starting any new workout, including the YogaFit workouts. You might occasionally feel sensations that are mildly uncomfortable as your body adjusts to a new workout or pose, and this is fine, but if the discomfort turns to pain cease the workout or pose immediately. Don't wait to adjust to the pain or for the pain to subside. Finally, allow yourself to rest when you need to. Do what you need to do to enjoy your workout session; this will keep you coming back.

BEFORE YOU START

As you learned in part I, a successful YogaFit practice is more than a workout—it's an experience for the mind and body that leads to greater health and joy. But to realize these benefits, you need to prepare yourself adequately and remember that yoga is more about the journey than the destination. Some key points should help you move in the right direction.

Familiarize yourself with the poses.   Take time to get familiar with the poses described in part II. The format of the workouts in this chapter are designed to help you remember how to do the poses, but full descriptions of the poses and their modifications are not included here. It's one thing to know the names of the poses and how they're supposed to look; it's another to understand how to make them fit your body and how to safely transition from one to the next.

Move controlled and consciously from pose to pose.
When performing a workout, observe your body without judgment, realizing that each body has its limits. When you need a break, move into the Child's Pose for a few breaths. Listen to your body; only you know what is good for you on any given day. Also, understand that your body will be tight in certain areas and more flexible in others. One side of your body will be more flexible than the other, and one side of your body will be stronger than the other. Observe and learn. Your YogaFit sessions should help you even out imbalances.

Be patient and consistent.   Often, you can accomplish certain poses only after practicing them regularly for a while. One of the beautiful moments in yoga is when you find yourself in a pose that you could not do in previous workouts. But never force a pose; never push yourself beyond your limits.

YogaFit is best practiced three to five times a week for 30 to 60 minutes each. Make time for your routine, and you'll soon notice a difference in the way you feel. You'll also learn that there is no "bad" or "wrong" YogaFit practice as long as you go at your own pace, breathe effectively, and allow yourself to experience how each pose feels at each moment. Remember, any movement is good movement as long as it is safe movement.

Learn that each practice is a reward in itself.   If you see each YogaFit session as its own reward you'll feel better without the risk of burning out or getting bored. Remember the YogaFit Essence and "let go of your expectations" each time you come to your mat. If you do, you'll be grateful for any shift or improvement, and you'll never leave your mat disappointed or feeling that you wasted your time. Make YogaFit your companion for life—it can help you achieve all your goals, not just the physical ones.

Important Reminders

- *Sun Salutations and Modified Sun Salutations* are the series of 12 poses described on page 32 in chapter 4. This series can be done on or off the knees, depending on your strength and stability. In the following workouts, warm up in Valley I with the modified version first, then progress to the full version as appropriate for your body, performing two to four sets (or more as your strength and fitness level increase).

- The *Flow Series*, or the bottom half of Sun Salutations (p. 32), can be done on or off the knees, depending on your strength and stability.

- Always start any series with the same foot. Repeat each series on the opposite side before moving on.

- As mentioned in Principles of Forward and Backward Bends (p. 105), the Swan Dive (see photos A-C) and Reverse Swan Dive (see photos D-F) are always the transition between the Standing Forward Fold and upright standing poses in workouts or series. Keep your knees bent, spine straight, and arms out to the side as you go either up or down. Avoid reaching directly forward with your arms because this increases the lever length and might strain your lower back (see SPA 7 on p. 7).

- Always begin with three to five minutes of deep breathing and then maintain a deep breath throughout, until the Final Relaxation phase.

- Breathing techniques and locks (p. 21) can be added where appropriate.

- Rest when you need to. We recommend the Child's Pose when resting, but you may use any pose that feels right to you.

YOGAFIT WORKOUTS

The workouts here vary in length and level of difficulty. Some are for beginners and others for people who have experience with YogaFit or who are in excellent physical condition. We group the workouts into four kinds.

- *Beginning YogaFit*—This short, less-intense workout for beginning students can be modified easily for special conditions. Those with more experience may come back to Beginning YogaFit when they need a restorative or healing practice session.

- *Flex and Flow*—This is a slightly longer beginner to intermediate workout that combines repetitive movement with static holds. It's a great total body workout that will make you sweat.

- *YogaCore*—Ready for a challenge? This longer workout targets your midsection, including your glutes and lower back, for muscular power and stamina. You'll do plenty of stretching and balance work as well.

- *Power YogaFit*—This workout is the most physically demanding we offer, with more complex sequences and additional Flow Series to increase heat and intensity. This workout is for healthy and experienced people looking to take their physical practice to the next level.

No matter what your experience or fitness level, start with the Beginning YogaFit workout to familiarize yourself with YogaFit and introduce your body and mind to the new format. Afterward, experiment with the other three workouts until you find one in which you feel challenged, yet successful. Stick with one, or vary your workout regularly, depending on what you need personally and physically. Following the workouts, the section called Taking Your Workout to the Next Level (p. 237) shows you how to progress by altering your workouts so that you always have a place to go as you improve and desire more from each practice.

Swan Dive

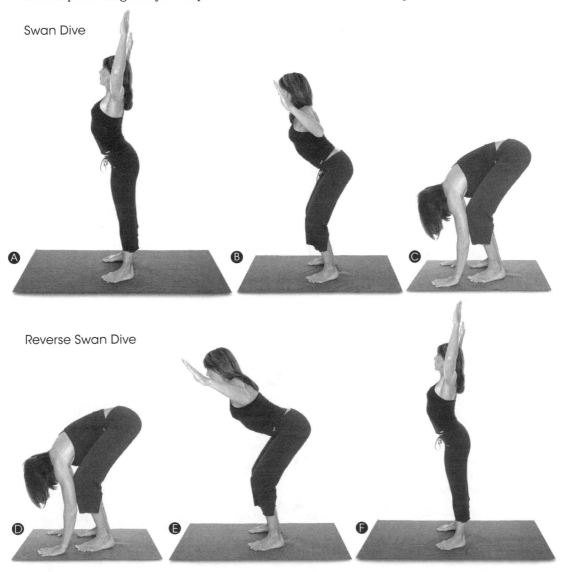

Reverse Swan Dive

Warm-Up

As you learned in chapter 4, a YogaFit session is based on the Three Mountains format and includes a warm-up, workout, and cool-down. This format ensures effective, safe, and consistent progression in every YogaFit workout. Just as it is important for the workout as a whole to be balanced, it is important for the warm-up be balanced. By targeting every major muscle group in your warm-up and moving the joints through their natural range of motion, you prepare your body to move into the workout phase of Mountain II.

Use one of these two balanced, comprehensive warm-ups to prepare for Mountain II. The first begins lying down and is effective for beginners, evening workouts, or even midday workouts when your mind is wandering and you need extra help centering. The second warm-up begins standing up—a great way to start the day or to begin a more vigorous practice.

Standard Lying Down Warm-Up

Relaxation on back (same as Final Relaxation, p. 196)		• 3-5 minutes of deep breathing.
Knees to Chest (p. 182)		• Hold one ham-string, and extend one leg at a time above the mat. Alternate legs. • Repeat 5-10 times, flowing with your breath.
Bridge (p. 140)		• Repeat 2-3 times, flowing with your breath. • Inhale as you lift; exhale as you lower your back to the mat.
Ab Work (p. 54)		• Repeat 5-6 times.
Knees to Chest (p. 182)		• Hold one hamstring and extend one leg at a time above the mat. Alternate legs. • Repeat 5-10 times, flowing with your breath.
Flowing Bridge (p. 140)		• Inhale as you lift; exhale as you lower your back to the mat. • Repeat 2-3 times, flowing with your breath.

Cat and Cow (p. 128)		• Repeat 5-10 times.
Spinal Balance (p. 56)		• Repeat 5-10 times.
Child's Pose (p. 164)		• Pause to check in.
Modified Flow Series (p. 32)	• Repeat 5-10 times. • Omit Cobra; instead push straight back into Child's Pose from Kneeling Plank.	
1. *Child's Pose* (p. 164)		• Sink hips toward heels.
2. *Kneeling Plank* (p. 40)		• Draw forward with a neutral spine.
3. *Kneeling Crocodile* (p. 42)		• Lower your upper body while lifting your abdominals.
4. *Child's Pose* (p. 164)		• Draw back, moving from your core.

Standard Standing Warm-Up

Mountain Pose (p. 66)		• 3-5 minutes of deep breathing.
Moonflowers (p. 68)		• Repeat 5-10 times.
Sunflowers (p. 70)		• Repeat 5-10 times.
Chair Flow (p. 88)		• Inhale with arms overhead; exhale sitting back into Chair. • Repeat 5 or more times.
Swan Dive and Reverse Swan Dive (p. 203)		• Bend knees and hinge from the hips, bringing hands to the floor. Reverse the Swan Dive by bending the knees and returning to Mountain Pose with a straight spine. • Keep arms out to the sides versus reaching forward. • Repeat 5 or more times.
Downward-Facing Dog (p. 108)		• Repeat 10 times with alternating heel press.
Child's Pose (p. 164)		• Hold for 5 breaths.

Cat and Cow (p. 128)		• Repeat 10-15 times.
Spinal Balance (p. 56)		• Repeat 5-10 times.
Modified Flow Series (p. 32)	• Omit Cobra; instead push straight back into Child's Pose from Kneeling Plank. • Repeat 5-10 times.	
1. *Child's Pose* (p. 164)		• Sink hips toward heels.
2. *Kneeling Plank* (p. 40)		• Draw forward with a neutral spine.
3. *Kneeling Crocodile* (p. 42)		• Lower upper body while lifting abdominals.
4. *Child's Pose* (p. 164)		• Draw back, moving from the core.
Downward-Facing Dog (p. 108)		• Hold for 5 breaths.
Reverse Swan Dive to Mountain Pose (p. 203 and p. 66)		• Bend knees and return to Mountain Pose with a straight spine. • Keep arms out to the sides versus reaching forward.

Beginning YogaFit

Beginning YogaFit is a fluid 45-minute total body workout appropriate for most healthy beginners of any age. Beginning YogaFit is a great place to learn the basic elements if you are brand new to yoga.

Mountain I: Warm-Up		
Standard Lying Down Warm-Up (see p. 204)		
Valley I: Sun Salutations		
Sun Salutations (p. 33)	• Repeat 2-4 times.	
1. *Mountain Pose* (p. 66)		• Stand with feet hip-width apart. • Establish a strong base.
2. *Standing Forward Fold* (p. 106)		• Swan Dive into the pose. • Place hands firmly on floor.
3. *Crescent Lunge or Kneeling Lunge* (p. 166)	*or*	• Reach back with one foot, maintaining alignment with hip.
4. *Downward- Facing Dog* (p. 108) *or Child's Pose* (p. 164)	*or*	• Press back, hinging from the hips.
5. *Plank or Kneeling Plank* (p. 40)	*or*	• Draw forward with a neutral spine.
6. *Crocodile or Kneeling Crocodile* (p. 42)	*or*	• Lower upper body while lifting abdominals.

7. *Upward-Facing Dog* (p. 46) *or Cobra* (p. 44)	*or*	• Lift and open the heart. • Lenthen out of lower back.
8. *Downward- Facing Dog* (p. 108) *or Child's Pose* (p. 164)	*or*	• Press back, hinging from the hips.
9. *Crescent Lunge or Kneeling Lunge* (p. 166)	*or*	• Step forward, stacking knee over ankle.
10. *Standing Forward Fold* (p. 106)		• Engage core. • Use Reverse Swan Dive to return to Mountain.
11. *Mountain Pose* (p. 66)		• Check in with your body and breath.
12. *Chair* (p. 88)		• Relax shoulders back and down. • Keep elbows soft. • Sit back, shifting weight to heels.

Mountain II: Work

Hold poses for 3-5 breaths unless otherwise noted.

Standing Lateral Flexion (p. 74)		• Repeat on both sides.

(continued)

Beginning YogaFit *(continued)*

Standing Chest Expansion with Forward Fold (p. 116)		
Warrior Series	• Repeat series on both sides.	
1. Warrior I (p. 76)		• Press back foot flat to floor. • Square shoulders with front of mat. • Point tailbone towards floor.
2. Warrior II (p. 78)		• Face long edge of mat. • Stack forward knee over ankle.
3. Triangle (p. 82)		• Maintain neutral spine.
4. Mountain Pose (p. 66)		• Check in with your body and breath.

Valley II: Upright Standing Balance

Tree (p. 96)		• Hold for 5-10 breaths. • Switch sides.

Mountain III: Cool-Down

Hold poses for 5-10 breaths unless otherwise noted.		
Child's Pose (p. 164)		• Sink hips toward heels.

Seated Straddle Splits (p. 126)		• Point knees and toes up. • Practice Sinking Breath.
Butterfly (p. 176)		• Soften toward floor. • Avoid pulling feet. • Practice Sinking Breath.
Tabletop (p. 50)		• Roll shoulders back and down before lifting. • Stack joints.
Knees to Chest (p. 182)		• Soften and relax.
Dead Bug (p. 184)		• Keep tailbone on floor.
Supine Spinal Twist (p. 158)		• Breathe deeply, allowing gravity to guide you into the pose.
Final Relaxation (p. 196)		• Let go of any remaining tension. • Stay for as long as time allows.

Flex and Flow

Flex and Flow is a one-hour, intermediate-level workout that fuses strength training with total body stretching. The "flex" refers to isometric holds in poses aimed at strengthening and toning your major muscle groups. The "flow" refers to a smooth and fluid series of poses that acts to counterbalance the extensive muscle contracting. This workout alternates flex with flow, simultaneously providing your body with challenge and release.

Mountain I: Warm-Up		
Standard Lying Down Warm-Up (see p. 204)		
Valley I: Sun Salutations		
Sun Salutations (p. 33)	• Repeat 2-4 times.	
1. *Mountain Pose* (p. 66)		• Stand with feet hip-width apart. • Establish a strong base.
2. *Standing Forward Fold* (p. 106)		• Swan Dive into the pose. • Place hands firmly on floor.
3. *Crescent Lunge or Kneeling Lunge* (p. 166)	*or*	• Reach back with one foot, maintaining alignment with hip.
4. *Downward- Facing Dog* (p. 108) *or Child's Pose* (p. 164)	*or*	• Press back, hinging from the hips.
5. *Plank or Kneeling Plank* (p. 40)	*or*	• Draw forward with a neutral spine.

6. *Crocodile or Kneeling Crocodile* (p. 42)	*or*	• Lower upper body while lifting abdominals.
7. *Upward-Facing Dog* (p. 46) *or Cobra* (p. 44)	*or*	• Lift and open the heart. • Lenthen out of lower back.
8. *Downward- Facing Dog* (p. 108) *or Child's Pose* (p. 164)	*or*	• Press back, hinging from the hips.
9. *Crescent Lunge or Kneeling Lunge* (p. 166)	*or*	• Step forward, stacking knee over ankle.
10. *Standing Forward Fold* (p. 106)		• Engage core. • Use Reverse Swan Dive to return to Mountain.
11. *Mountain Pose* (p. 66)		• Check in with your body and breath.
12. *Chair* (p. 88)		• Relax shoulders back and down. • Keep elbows soft. • Sit back, shifting weight to heels.

(continued)

Flex and Flow *(continued)*

Mountain II: Work		
Hold poses for 3-5 breaths unless otherwise noted.		
Down Dog Leg Lifts		• In Downward-Facing Dog (p. 108), alternate lifting one leg at a time straight up and back. • Hold each side for 3-5 breaths, then flow from side to side 5 times with your breath.
One-Arm Down Dog		• In Downward-Facing Dog (p. 108), place one hand behind your back. • Repeat on both sides.
Child's Pose (p. 164)		• Sink hips toward heels.
Camel (p. 134)		• Lift heart and lengthen out of lower back. • Practice Expanding Breath.
Plank Push-Up Series	• First time through the series, hold each pose for 3 breaths. Switch sides. Then, alternate sides 3 times, flowing one breath per movement. • Eliminate the one-legged options as desired.	
1. *Three-Legged Downward-Facing Dog* (p. 108)		• From Downward-Facing Dog, lift one leg high to the sky.
2. *Upward-Facing Dog* (p. 46)		• From one-legged Plank, place just the tops of both feet on the mat and draw your chest forward.

3. *Plank Push-Up* (p. 40)		• From Upward-Facing Dog, return to Plank and lower to Crocodile for a "push-up."
4. *Downward-Facing Dog* (p. 108)		• From Crocodile, press back to Plank and return to Downward-Facing Dog.
Crescent Lunge (p. 166)		• Repeat on both sides.
Downward-Facing Dog (p. 108)		• Spread fingers wide. • Lengthen spine. • Bend knees as necessary to lessen intensity.
Sunflowers (p. 70)		• Repeat 5 times.
Sun Pose (p. 72)		• Practice Three-Part Breath.
Chair (p. 88)		• Relax shoulders back and down. • Keep elbows soft. • Sit back, shifting weight to heels.
Twisting Chair (p. 150)		• Hold pose for 3-5 breaths on each side. • Alternate sides flowing with the breath 5 times.

(continued)

Flex and Flow *(continued)*

Standing Lateral Flexion (p. 74)		• Repeat on both sides.
Warrior II Flow (p. 78)		• Hold Warrior II for 3-5 breaths. Then, bend and straighten the forward leg. • Repeat 5 times. • Switch sides.
Standing Straddle Splits (p. 122)		• For an optional chest expansion, interlace your fingers behind your back and straighten your arms, lifting your knuckles toward the sky.
Side Angle Flow Series	• Turn toward back foot and repeat series on other side. • Upon completion, turn again to face front of mat.	
1. Side Angle (p. 84)		• Sink through hips. • Avoid sinking into bottom hand or shoulder.
2. Side Angle Arm Circles (p. 84)		• Circle top arm by reaching forward, down and around, 5 times with the breath.
3. Triangle (p. 82)		• Maintain neutral spine.

4. *Pyramid* (p. 114)		• For an optional chest expansion, interlace your fingers behind your back and straighten your arms, lifting your knuckles toward the sky.
5. *Twisting Triangle* (p. 148)		• Rotate without rounding your back. • Let go of expectations. • Stay in the present moment.
6. *Pyramid* (p. 114)		• Keep hips square with front of mat. • Practice Sinking Breath to stretch entire back of body.
7. *Reverse Swan Dive from Pyramid* (p. 203 and 114)		• From Pyramid, return to standing by maintaining a strong core, keeping a straight spine, and extending arms out to each side.
Standing Forward Fold (p. 106)		• Engage your core. • Use Reverse Swan Dive to return to Mountain.
Downward-Facing Dog (p. 108)		• Pedal feet 10 times.
Flow Series (p. 32)	• First time through, hold each pose for 3-5 breaths. Then, as usual, flow with the breath. • Perform Modified Flow Series instead, if necessary. • Repeat 3 times.	
1. *Downward-Facing Dog* (p. 108)		• Spread fingers wide. • Lengthen spine. • Bend knees as necessary to lessen intensity.

(continued)

Flex and Flow *(continued)*

2. Plank (p. 40)		• Draw forward with a neutral spine.
3. *Crocodile* (p. 42)		• Lower upper body while lifting abdominals.
4. *Upward-Facing Dog* (p. 46)		• Lift and open the heart. • Lengthen out of lower back.
5. *Downward-Facing Dog* (p. 108)		• Spread fingers wide. • Lengthen spine. • Bend knees as necessary to lessen intensity.
Standing Backbend (p. 130)		• Establish a strong base. • Lift out of lower back.
Standing Chest Expansion with Forward Fold (p. 116)		• For lower back discomfort or injury, remain standing upright.

Valley II: Upright Standing Balance

Dancer (p. 102)		• Hold for 5-10 breaths. • Switch sides.

Mountain III: Cool-Down

Hold poses for 5-10 breaths unless otherwise noted.

Ab Work (p. 54)		• Exhale as you lift, inhale as you release.

Boat Flow (p. 58)		• In Boat, lean back creating more space between chest and thighs. Exhale back to Boat, inhale, open. Move arms as if rowing a boat. • Repeat 5 to 10 times.
Big-Toe Wide Boat (p. 60)		• Hold for 5-10 breaths.
Tabletop Flow (p. 50)		• In Tabletop, lift and extend one leg. • Switch sides. • Option to bend elbows for tricep push-ups or keep both feet on the floor. • Repeat 5 times.
Butterfly (p. 176)		• Soften toward floor. • Avoid pulling feet. • Practice Sinking Breath.
Turkish Twist (p. 156)		• Inhale and lengthen. • Exhale and rotate.
Dead Bug (p. 184)		• Keep tailbone on floor.
Bridge (p. 140)		• Inhale as you lift into Bridge, exhale as you lower your back to the mat. • Repeat 3-5 times.
Ab Work (p. 54)		• Bring opposite shoulder, not elbow, to opposite knee.

(continued)

Flex and Flow *(continued)*

Bridge (p. 140)		• Inhale as you lift into Bridge, exhale as you lower your back to the mat. • Repeat 3-5 times.
Upside-Down Pigeon (p. 178)		• Breathe deeply to release tension.
Butterfly (p. 176)		• Soften toward floor. • Avoid pulling feet. • Practice Sinking Breath.
Shoulderstand and Plow or Legs Up Wall (pp. 192, 190, and 188)	*and* *or*	• Practice inversions for greater mental and physical well-being. • Keep head in line with spine. • Hold for 5-10 breaths.
Supine Spinal Twist (p. 158)		• Breathe deeply, allowing gravity to guide you into the pose.
Fish (p. 194)		• Follows inversions as a counterpose to open throat and chest.
Knees to Chest (p. 182)		• Hold hamstrings and relax to release back.
Final Relaxation (p. 196)		• Let go of any remaining tension. • Stay for as long as time allows.

YogaCore

YogaCore is a 60- to 75-minute hybrid yoga–fitness workout for intermediate and experienced practitioners. YogaCore targets the midsection and additional muscle groups surrounding and assisting the midsection, including the lower back. This workout incorporates more repetition for muscular endurance and involves holding poses for increased strength.

Mountain I: Warm-Up		
Standard Lying Down Warm-Up (see p. 204)		
Valley I: Sun Salutations		
Sun Salutations (p. 36)	• Repeat 2-4 times.	
1. Mountain Pose (p. 66)		• Stand with feet hip-width apart. • Establish a strong base.
2. Standing Forward Fold (p. 106)		• Swan Dive into the pose. • Place hands firmly on floor.
3. Crescent Lunge or Kneeling Lunge (p. 166)	or	• Reach back with one foot, maintaining alignment with hip.
4. Downward-Facing Dog (p. 108) or Child's Pose (p. 164)	or	• Press back, hinging from the hips.
5. Plank or Kneeling Plank (p. 40)	or	• Draw forward with a neutral spine.

(continued)

YogaCore *(continued)*

6. *Crocodile or Kneeling Crocodile* (p. 42)	*or*	• Lower upper body while lifting abdominals.
7. *Upward-Facing Dog or Cobra* (p. 44)	*or*	• Lift and open the heart. • Lenthen out of lower back.
8. *Downward- Facing Dog* (p. 108) *or Child's Pose* (p. 164)	*or*	• Press back, hinging from the hips.
9. *Crescent Lunge or Kneeling Lunge* (p. 166)	*or*	• Step forward, stacking knee over ankle.
10. *Standing Forward Fold* (p. 106)		• Engage core. • Use Reverse Swan Dive to return to Mountain.
11. *Mountain Pose* (p. 66)		• Check in with your body and breath.
12. *Chair* (p. 88)		• Relax shoulders back and down. • Keep elbows soft. • Sit back, shifting weight to heels.

Mountain II: Work

Hold poses for 3-5 breaths unless otherwise noted.

Sun Squats (p. 72)		• From Sun Pose, inhale while straightening both legs and bring arms overhead; exhale returning to Sun Pose. • Repeat 5-10 times.
Mountain Pose (p. 66)		• Check in with your body and breath.
Standing Forward Fold (p. 106)		• Engage core. • Use Reverse Swan Dive to return to Mountain.
Plank (p. 40)		• From Standing Forward Fold, step, hop, or float back into Plank.
Side Plank Lifts (p. 52)		• From Kneeling Side Plank, lift and lower the extended leg, keeping your toes flexed. • Repeat 5-10 times on each side.
Down Dog Leg Lifts (p. 108)		• From Downward-Facing Dog, lift one leg at a time straight up and back. • Repeat 5 times on each side.
Repeater Crescent Lunges (p. 166)		• From Crescent Lunge, repeatedly pull knee up to chest and return to starting position. • Repeat 5-10 times on each side.

(continued)

YogaCore *(continued)*

Plank With Leg Lifts (p. 40)		• In Plank or Kneeling Plank, lift one leg at a time away from the floor, maintaining a strong core center. • Hold for 5 breaths on each side.
Standing Forward Fold (p. 106)		• Engage core. • Use Reverse Swan Dive to return to Mountain.
Mountain Pose (p. 66)		• Check in with your body and breath.
Chair (p. 88)		• Relax shoulders back and down. • Keep elbows soft. • Sit back, shifting weight to heels.
Standing Backbend (p. 130)		• Establish a strong base. • Lift out of lower back.
Standing Chest Expansion With Forward Fold (p. 116)		• For lower back discomfort or injury, remain upright.
Downward-Facing Dog (p. 108)		• Spread fingers wide. • Lengthen spine. • Bend knees as necessary to lessen intensity.
Valley II: Upright Standing Balance		
Standing Balance Pigeon (p. 100)		• Hold for 5-10 breaths. • Switch sides.

Standing Spinal Twist (p. 152)		• Hold for 5-10 breaths. • Switch sides.

Mountain III: Cool-Down

Hold poses for 5-10 breaths unless otherwise noted.

Downward-Facing Dog (p. 108)		• Spread fingers wide. • Lengthen spine. • Bend knees as necessary to lessen intensity.
Child's Pose (p. 164)		• Sink hips toward heels.
Locust (p. 136)		• Option to use Superman (p. 136)
Bow (p. 138)		• Watch for signs of struggle. • Create tension without stress.
Child's Pose (p. 164)		• Sink hips toward heels.
Boat (p. 58)		• Lift your chest to align your spine.
Tabletop (p. 50)		• Roll shoulders back and down before lifting. • Stack joints.
Seated Forward Fold (124)		• Draw forward using lower abdominals. • Practice feeling, not forcing.
Seated Straddle Splits (126)		• Point knees and toes up. • Practice Sinking Breath.
Turkish Twist (p. 156)		• Inhale and lengthen. • Exhale and rotate.

(continued)

YogaCore *(continued)*

Seated Spinal Twist (p. 154)		• Sit tall. • Relax shoulders back and down. • Rotate from bottom to top.
Butterfly (p. 176)		• Soften toward floor. • Avoid pulling feet. • Practice Sinking Breath.
Knees to Chest (p. 182)		• Hold hamstrings and relax to release back.
Ab Work (p. 54)		• Bring opposite shoulder, not elbow, to opposite knee.
Bridge (p. 140)		• Place feet hip-width apart. • Slide shoulders away from ears before lifting.
Shoulderstand and Plow or Legs Up Wall (pp. 192, 190, and 188)	*and* *or*	• Practice inversions for greater mental and physical well-being. • Keep head in line with spine. • Hold for 5-10 breaths.
Fish (p. 194)		• Follows inversions as a counterpose to open throat and chest.
Final Relaxation (p. 196)		• Let go of any remaining tension. • Stay for as long as time allows.

Power YogaFit

Power YogaFit is a vigorous 75-minute workout for those who are advanced practitioners of YogaFit or who are in very good physical health. Power YogaFit moves faster for more cardiovascular benefits and also yields increased strength, endurance, balance, and flexibility.

Mountain I: Warm-Up		
Standard Standing Warm-Up (see p. 206)		
Valley I: Sun Salutations		
Sun Salutations (p. 33)	• Repeat 2-4 times.	
1. *Mountain Pose* (p. 66)		• Stand with feet hip-width apart. • Establish a strong base.
2. *Standing Forward Fold* (p. 106)		• Swan Dive into the pose. • Place hands firmly on floor.
3. *Crescent Lunge or Kneeling Lunge* (p. 166)	*or*	• Reach back with one foot, maintaining alignment with hip.
4. *Downward-Facing Dog* (p. 108) *or Child's Pose* (p. 164)	*or*	• Press back, hinging from the hips.
5. *Plank or Kneeling Plank* (p. 40)	*or*	• Draw forward with a neutral spine.

(continued)

Power YogaFit (continued)

6. Crocodile or Kneeling Crocodile (p. 42)	*or*	• Lower upper body while lifting abdominals.
7. Upward-Facing Dog (p. 46) or Cobra (p. 44)	*or*	• Lift and open the heart. • Lenthen out of lower back.
8. Downward- Facing Dog (p. 108) or Child's Pose (p. 164)	*or*	• Press back, hinging from the hips.
9. Crescent Lunge or Kneeling Lunge (p. 166)	*or*	• Step forward, stacking knee over ankle.
10. Standing Forward Fold (p. 106)		• Engage core. • Use Reverse Swan Dive to return to Mountain.
11. Mountain Pose (p. 66)		• Check in with your body and breath.
12. Chair (p. 88)		• Relax shoulders back and down. • Keep elbows soft. • Sit back, shifting weight to heels.

Mountain II: Work

Hold poses for 3-5 breaths unless otherwise noted.

Downward-Facing Dog (p. 108)		• Note that the transition into Standing Forward Fold can be made by stepping, hopping, or "floating" the feet between the hands.
Standing Forward Fold (p. 106)		• Engage your core. • Use Reverse Swan Dive to return to Mountain.
Mountain Pose (p. 66)		• Check in with your body and breath.
Twisting Chair Flow Series	• Repeat 2-4 times, alternating sides.	
1. *Twisting Chair* (p. 150)		• Inhale arms overhead; exhale easing into Twisting Chair.
2. *Standing Forward Fold* (p. 106)		• Exhale into forward fold with bent legs.
3. *Reverse Swan Dive* (p. 203)		• Keep knees bent and spine straight.
4. *Twisting Chair* (p. 150)		• Keep knees together. • Lift heart to lengthen spine before rotating.

(continued)

Power YogaFit *(continued)*

Flow Series (p. 32)	• Repeat 5-10 times.	
1. *Downward-Facing Dog* (p. 108)		• Press back, hinging from the hips.
2. *Plank* (p. 40)		• Draw forward with a neutral spine.
3. *Crocodile* (p. 42)		• Lower upper body while lifting abdominals.
4. *Upward-Facing Dog* (p. 46)		• Lift and open the heart. • Lengthen out of lower back.
5. *Downward-Facing Dog* (p. 108)		• Press back, hinging from the hips.
6. *Plank* (p. 40)		• Draw forward with a neutral spine.
Twisting Lunge Flow Series	• Repeat on both sides.	
1. *Downward-Facing Dog* (p. 108)		• Press back, hinging from the hips.
2. *Crescent Lunge* (p. 166)		• Step forward, stacking knee over ankle.
3. *Twisting Lunge* (p. 146)		• Follow your breath into the rotation. • Let go of judgment.
4. *Downward-Facing Dog* (p. 108)		• Press back, hinging from the hips.

Flow Series (p. 32)	(See *Flow Series* earlier in this workout)	• Repeat 3-5 times.
Downward-Facing Dog (p. 108)		• Spread fingers wide. • Lengthen spine. • Bend knees as necessary to lessen intensity.
Side Angle Flow Series	• Repeat on each side.	
1. *Warrior I* (p. 76)		• Press back foot flat to floor. • Square shoulders with front of mat. • Point tailbone towards floor.
2. *Warrior II* (p. 78)		• Face long edge of mat. • Stack forward knee over ankle.
3. *Reverse Warrior* (p. 80)		• Remember to side bend, not back bend.
4. *Side Angle* (p. 84)		• Sink through hips. • Avoid sinking into bottom hand or shoulder.
Flow Series (p. 32)	(See *Flow Series* earlier in this workout)	• Repeat 3-5 times.
Downward-Facing Dog (p. 108)		• Spread fingers wide. • Lengthen spine. • Bend knees as necessary to lessen intensity.
Prayer Twisting Flow Series	• Repeat on each side.	
1. *Crescent Lunge* (p. 166)		• For less intensity, place fingers on floor or drop back knee.

(continued)

Power YogaFit *(continued)*

2. *Prayer Twisting Lunge* (p. 146)		• Practice dynamic tension and surrender.
3. *Standing Straddle Splits* (p. 122)		• Gently contract your thighs. • Place feet flat on floor. • Lift shoulders away from ears.
4. *Crescent Lunge (p. 166)*		• For less intensity, place fingers on floor or drop back knee.
5. *Downward-Facing Dog* (p. 108)		• Spread fingers wide. • Lengthen spine. • Bend knees as necessary to lessen intensity.
Standing Forward Fold (p. 106)		• Engage your core. • Use Reverse Swan Dive to return to Mountain.
Standing Backbend (p. 130)		• Establish a strong base. • Lift out of lower back.
Standing Forward Fold (p. 106)		• Engage your core. • Use Reverse Swan Dive to return to Mountain.
Mountain Pose (p. 66)		• Check in with your body and breath.

Triangle Series	• Repeat series on both sides.	
1. *Triangle* (p. 82)		• Maintain neutral spine.
2. *Pyramid* (p. 114)		• Keep hips square with front of mat. • Practice Sinking Breath to stretch back of body.
3. *Twisting Triangle* (p. 148)		• Rotate without rounding back. • Let go of expectations. • Stay in the present moment.
4. *Pyramid* (p. 114)		• Keep hips square with front of mat. • Practice Sinking Breath to stretch back of body.
5. *Standing Forward Fold* (p. 106)		• Engage your core. • Use Reverse Swan Dive to return to Mountain.
Standing Straddle Splits (p. 122)		• Gently contract your thighs. • Place feet flat on floor. • Lift shoulders away from ears.
Standing Forward Fold (p. 106)		• Engage your core. • Use Reverse Swan Dive to return to Mountain.
Dolphin/Plank Flow Series	• Repeat series 3-5 times.	
1. *Plank* (p. 40)		• Draw forward with a neutral spine.
2. *Child's Pose* (p. 164)		• Sink hips toward heels.

(continued)

Power YogaFit *(continued)*

3. Dolphin (p. 110)		• From Child's Pose, inhale bringing chin over thumbs, exhale pressing back to Dolphin.
Downward-Facing Dog (p. 108)		• Spread fingers wide. • Lengthen spine. • Bend knees as necessary to lessen intensity.
Three-Legged Downward-Facing Dog (p. 108)		• From Downward-Facing Dog, lift one leg high to the sky. • Repeat on each side.
Side Plank (p. 52)		• Stack wrists and shoulders. • For shoulder injuries or discomfort, place knee on floor below hip.
Child's Pose (p. 164)		• Sink hips toward heels.

Valley II: Upright Standing Balance

Hold poses for 5-10 breaths unless otherwise noted.

Warrior III (p. 90)		• Option to transition directly from Warrior III to Eagle by bringing the elevated leg forward and wrapping it around the standing leg. • Bend the standing leg and engage root lock (chapter 3) for a safer transition.

Eagle (p. 98)		• Gently wrap your body in a hug. • Breathe deeply.

Mountain III: Cool-Down

Hold poses for 5-10 breaths unless otherwise noted.

Seated Forward Fold (p. 124)		• Draw forward using your lower abdominals.
Tabletop (p. 50)		• Option to flow from Tabletop to Boat 3 times.
Boat (p. 58)		• Option to flow from Tabletop to Boat 3 times.
Ab Work (p. 54)		• Bring opposite shoulder, not elbow, to opposite knee.
Seated Spinal Twist (p. 154)		• Sit tall. • Relax shoulders back and down. • Rotate from bottom to top.
Turkish Twist (p. 156)		• Inhale and lengthen. • Exhale and rotate.
Dead Bug (p. 184)		• Keep tailbone on floor.
Bridge (p. 140) or Wheel (p. 142)	or	• Expect increased energy and alertness. • Practice expanding breath.

(continued)

Power YogaFit *(continued)*

Big Toe Hold (p. 186)		• This pose combines strength, flexibility, effort, and surrender. • Hold each phase for 5 breaths.
Knees to Chest (p. 182)		• Hold hamstrings and relax to release back.
Shoulderstand and Plow or Legs Up Wall (pp. 192, 190, and 188)	*and* *or*	• Practice inversions for greater mental and physical well-being. • Keep head in line with spine. • Hold for 5-10 breaths.
Fish (p. 194)		• Follows inversions as a counterpose to open throat and chest.
Final Relaxation (p. 196)		• Let go of any remaining tension. • Stay for as long as time allows.

Taking Your Workout to the Next Level

There's always a next step in YogaFit. There's no such thing as mastering a pose, no matter how basic it seems, because every day your body is different, and your circumstances are different, ensuring that you'll always find a new place to go.

However, as you become stronger and more flexible, you might want more from your practice. Whether you stay with the Beginning YogaFit format, or progress to Power Yoga, you can always make any format more challenging through simple modifications.

- Increase the number of Sun Salutations in Valley I.

- Hold Mountain II poses longer than three to five breaths. As long as you can maintain a steady, deep breath, without experiencing pain, you can stay as long as you like.

- Use the Flow Series (p. 32) in Mountains I and II. Add repetitions of this flow, on or off the knees, wherever you like to create more heat, increase your heart rate, and build strength.

- Hold Mountain III poses longer than 5 to 10 breaths. As long as you can maintain a steady, deep breath, without experiencing pain, you can stay as long as you like.

- Move through the poses with only one or two breaths in each pose for a more cardiovascular workout.

SPORT-SPECIFIC POSES

YogaFit was designed specifically for athletes and people interested in getting a good, total body–mind workout. Traditional exercise programs often overwork certain muscle groups or build muscle bulk unevenly. They tend to neglect training participants to breathe efficiently or to improve their mental game. YogaFit can be extremely helpful in counteracting some of the negative effects of these traditional programs and in expanding programs to focus on more than just muscular strength.

As an athlete, you can and will benefit from a regular YogaFit workout, but you might also want to complement your practice with sport-specific poses for strengthening, stretching, endurance, balance, focus, and relaxation. Use these poses either before or after your regular workout or training, or between weightlifting sets. These poses should improve your performance in your sport, reduce your risk of injury, and add to your overall enjoyment.

As always, before practicing any of the following poses, review part I as well as the corresponding pose pages in part II.

Swimming

Swimming and YogaFit have much in common in that both focus on moving and breathing rhythmically. For all levels of swimmers, YogaFit breathing is key—first, learning to unite the breath with movement in the water, and then practicing specific breathing techniques out of the water to improve concentration, breath control, and endurance. YogaFit poses can help balance the strength swimmers build in their upper bodies and shoulders with flexibility, for a healthier range of motion. Also, because swimming favors the upper body at the expense of the legs and core muscles, standing poses such as the Warrior poses and the Chair, along with abdominal work on the floor, can help your body maintain muscular balance.

Strength Focus		
Ab Work (p. 54)		• One breath per movement.
Locust or Superman (p. 136)	*or*	• Hold for 5-10 breaths.
Bow (p. 138)		• Hold for 5-10 breaths.
Incline Plank (p. 48)		• Hold for 5-10 breaths.
Warrior I (p. 76)		• Hold for 3-5 breaths.
Warrior II (p. 78)		• Hold for 3-5 breaths.

Warrior III (p. 90)		• Hold for 5-10 breaths.

Flexibility Focus

Standing Chest Expansion with Forward Fold (p. 116)		• Hold for 3-5 breaths.
Kneeling Shoulder Stretch (p. 170)		• Hold for 5-10 breaths.
Standing Backbend (p. 130)		• Hold for 5-10 breaths.
Camel (p. 134)		• Hold for 5-10 breaths.

Additional Practice

• Practice Three-Part breath (p. 22) and other breathing techniques for more efficient, focused, and intense workouts.

• Improve performance through meditation and visualization.

• Perform any standing balance poses (chapter 6).

Running

Because of the repetitive motion of the legs, running creates tightness in the hip flexors, hamstrings, and quads, often leading to lower back pain. Running also fails to strengthen the upper body or the abdominals. The YogaFit poses here serve as counterposes to offset runners' lower-body strength and to provide supplemental work to increase total body strength, endurance, and flexibility. Many runners find yoga keeps them running longer and faster, without the nagging injuries.

Strength Focus		
Ab Work (p. 54)		• One breath per movement.
Modified Flow Series (p. 32)	• One breath per movement. • Perform Flow Series instead (p. 32).	
1. Child's Pose (p. 164)		• Sink hips toward heels.
2. Kneeling Plank (p. 40)		• Draw forward with a neutral spine.
3. Kneeling Crocodile (p. 42)		• Lower upper body while lifting abdominals.
4. Cobra (p. 44)		• Lift and open the heart. • Lenthen out of lower back.
5. Child's Pose (p. 164)		• Sink hips toward heels.
Incline Plank (p. 48)		• Hold for 5-10 breaths.
Bow (p. 138)		• Hold for 5-10 breaths.

Flexibility Focus

Kneeling Lunge (p. 166)		• Hold for 5-10 breaths.
Quad Stretch (p. 168)		• Hold for 5-10 breaths.
Butterfly (p. 176)		• Hold for 5-10 breaths.
Upside-Down Pigeon (p. 178)		• Hold for 5-10 breaths.
Seated Forward Fold (p. 124)		• Hold for 5-10 breaths.

Additional Practice

• Practice Three-Part breath (p. 22) and other breathing techniques for more efficient, focused, and intense workouts.

• Improve performance through meditation and visualization.

• Perform any standing balance poses, especially Tree (p. 96) and Dancer (p. 102).

Cycling

Like running, cycling requires repetitive motion that shortens and tightens certain leg muscles while underusing others. Cycling also overstretches and underuses certain muscles in the upper back and abdomen, leading to postural alignment issues and, in some cases, back pain. In YogaFit, cyclists should focus on poses that counteract the seated and forward-reaching position they adopt in cycling; they should also do deep stretches that target their legs and hips. Practiced regularly, these poses help cyclists feel better longer, on and off the bike.

Strength Focus		
Ab Work (p. 54)		• One breath per movement.
Modified Flow Series (p. 32)	• One breath per movement. • Perform Flow Series instead (p. 32).	
1. *Child's Pose* (p. 164)		• Sink hips toward heels.
2. *Kneeling Plank* (p. 40)		• Draw forward with a neutral spine.
3. *Kneeling Crocodile* (p. 42)		• Lower upper body while lifting abdominals.
4. *Cobra* (p. 44)		• Lift and open the heart. • Lengthen out of lower back.
5. *Child's Pose* (p. 164)		• Sink hips toward heels.
Bridge (p. 140)		• Hold for 5-10 breaths.
Bow (p. 138)		• Hold for 5-10 breaths.

Flexibility Focus		
Kneeling Lunge (p. 166)		• Hold for 5-10 breaths.
Pyramid (p. 114)		• Hold for 3-5 breaths.
Frog (p. 174)		• Hold for 5-10 breaths.
Quad Stretch (p. 168)		• Hold for 5-10 breaths.
Butterfly (p. 176)		• Hold for 5-10 breaths.

Additional Practice

• Practice Three-Part breath (p. 22) and other breathing techniques for more efficient, focused, and intense workouts.

• Improve performance through meditation and visualization.

• Perform shoulder rolls.

• Perform any standing balance poses, especially Tree (p. 96) and Dancer (p. 102).

Golf

A common complaint among golfers is lower back pain. Golfers lean forward as they stand, which causes back strain, and they aggravate this strain by swinging in the same direction more than 100 times a round. Even just a few YogaFit poses to strengthen the back and rotate the spine in *both* directions can go a long way toward increasing power and decreasing tension for golfers. Improved concentration and relaxation through meditation and visualization can give a golfer the edge necessary to master what is largely a mental game.

Strength Focus		
Ab Work (p. 54)		• One breath per movement.
Modified Flow Series (p. 32)	• One breath per movement. • Perform Flow Series instead (p. 32).	
1. *Child's Pose* (p. 164)		• Sink hips toward heels.
2. *Kneeling Plank* (p. 40)		• Draw forward with a neutral spine.
3. *Kneeling Crocodile* (p. 42)		• Lower upper body while lifting abdominals.
4. *Cobra* (p. 44)		• Lift and open the heart. • Lengthen out of lower back.
5. *Child's Pose* (p. 164)		• Sink hips toward heels.
Bridge (p. 140)		• Hold for 5-10 breaths.

Flexibility Focus

Camel (p. 134)		• Hold for 5-10 breaths.
Kneeling Lunge (p. 166)		• Hold for 5-10 breaths.
Seated Spinal Twist (p. 154)		• Hold for 5-10 breaths.
Upside-Down Pigeon (p. 178)		• Hold for 5-10 breaths.

Additional Practice

• Practice Relaxation breath (p. 23) for focus and concentration.
• Improve mental game through meditation and visualization.
• Perform Standing Lateral Flexion (p. 74).
• Perform any twists (chapter 8).
• Perform any standing balance poses (chapter 6).
• Perform shoulder rolls and stretches.

Tennis

In tennis we favor one side of the body and place huge demands on the dominant shoulder, shortening our range of motion and creating other imbalances in the upper body and spine that can lead to pain and injury. Tennis also causes tightness in the hips and hamstrings, which can result in back pain. YogaFit poses help create length in both sides of the torso, rotate the spine in both directions for balance, and promote both strength and flexibility in and around the shoulders, which is critical for stability and a powerful serve.

Strength Focus		
Ab Work (p. 54)		• One breath per movement.
Modified Flow Series (p. 32)	• One breath per movement. • Perform Flow Series instead (p. 32).	
1. Child's Pose (p. 164)		• Sink hips toward heels.
2. Kneeling Plank (p. 40)		• Draw forward with a neutral spine.
3. Kneeling Crocodile (p. 42)		• Lower upper body while lifting abdominals.
4. Cobra (p. 44)		• Lift and open the heart. • Lengthen out of lower back.
5. Child's Pose (p. 164)		• Sink hips toward heels.
Downward-Facing Dog (p. 108)		• Hold for 3-5 breaths.
Bridge (p. 140)		• Hold for 5-10 breaths.

Flexibility Focus		
Standing Chest Expansion with Forward Fold (p. 116)		• Hold for 3-5 breaths.
Kneeling Shoulder Stretch (p. 170)		• Hold for 5-10 breaths.
Camel (p. 134)		• Hold for 5-10 breaths.
Upside-Down Pigeon (p. 178)		• Hold for 5-10 breaths.
Frog (p. 174)		• Hold for 5-10 breaths.
Seated Forward Fold (p. 124)		• Hold for 5-10 breaths.

Additional Practice

• Practice Relaxation breath (p. 23) for focus and concentration.
• Improve mental game through meditation and visualization.
• Perform Standing Lateral Flexion (p. 74).
• Perform any twists (chapter 8).
• Perform any standing balance poses (chapter 6).
• Perform shoulder rolls and stretches.

Baseball and Softball

Baseball and softball players favor one side of the body and tend to shorten their range of motion, creating imbalances that can lead to pain and injury. Softball and baseball cause tightness in the hips, quads, and hamstrings, so players might develop back pain. In addition, these games require a flexible torso, which can be developed and maintained through twists. Because these sports strongly favor a dominant side, YogaFit poses are necessary to prevent dramatic imbalances and to increase strength on the weaker side. Focusing on balancing right and left increases the strength of the whole body, making for better performance and less pain.

Strength Focus		
Ab Work (p. 54)		• One breath per movement.
Modified Flow Series (p. 32)	• One breath per movement. • Perform Flow Series instead (p. 32).	
1. Child's Pose (p. 164)		• Sink hips toward heels.
2. Kneeling Plank (p. 40)		• Draw forward with a neutral spine.
3. Kneeling Crocodile (p. 42)		• Lower upper body while lifting abdominals.
4. Cobra (p. 44)		• Lift and open the heart. • Lengthen out of lower back.
5. Child's Pose (p. 164)		• Sink hips toward heels.
Bow (p. 138)		• Hold for 5-10 breaths.
Bridge (p. 140)		• Hold for 5-10 breaths.

Flexibility Focus

Standing Chest Expansion with Forward Fold (p. 116)		• Hold for 3-5 breaths.
Kneeling Shoulder Stretch (p. 170)		• Hold for 5-10 breaths.
Camel (p. 134)		• Hold for 5-10 breaths.
Upside-Down Pigeon (p. 178)		• Hold for 5-10 breaths.
Frog (p. 174)		• Hold for 5-10 breaths.
Seated Forward Fold (p. 124)		• Hold for 5-10 breaths.

Additional Practice

• Practice Relaxation breath (p. 23) for focus and concentration.
• Improve mental game through meditation and visualization.
• Perform Standing Lateral Flexion (p. 74).
• Perform any twists (chapter 8).
• Perform any standing balance poses, especially Eagle (p. 98).
• Perform shoulder rolls and stretches.

Volleyball and Basketball

Volleyball and basketball are popular recreational sports, but over time they tend to demand more than the body can give, leading to shoulder and knee injuries. Whether players play for fun or competitively, they should balance the demands of these sports with yoga poses that stretch and strengthen their shoulders and back, stabilize their knees, and increase their core strength for jumps and lower back support. Athletes in these sports should also increase their cardiovascular endurance through breathing practices that strengthen the diaphragm.

Strength Focus		
Ab Work (p. 54)		• One breath per movement.
Modified Flow Series (p. 32)	• One breath per movement. • Perform Flow Series instead (p. 32).	
1. Child's Pose (p. 164)		• Sink hips toward heels.
2. Kneeling Plank (p. 40)		• Draw forward with a neutral spine.
3. Kneeling Crocodile (p. 42)		• Lower upper body while lifting abdominals.
4. Cobra (p. 44)		• Lift and open the heart. • Lengthen out of lower back.
5. Child's Pose (p. 164)		• Sink hips toward heels.
Bridge (p. 140)		• Hold for 5-10 breaths.
Warrior I (p. 76)		• Hold for 3-5 breaths.

Flexibility Focus		
Standing Chest Expansion With Forward Fold (p. 116)		• Hold for 3-5 breaths.
Camel (p. 134)		• Hold for 5-10 breaths.

Additional Practice

- Practice Three-Part breath (p. 22) and other breathing techniques for more efficient, focused, and intense workouts.
- Improve mental game through meditation and visualization.
- Perform Standing Lateral Flexion (p. 74).
- Perform any twists (chapter 8).
- Perform any standing balance poses, especially Eagle (p. 98).
- Perform shoulder rolls and stretches.

Skiing and Snowboarding

Balance is a primary focus for skiers and snowboarders, as is stretching the lower body, including the hips, quads, and hamstrings. As with all sports that overwork these muscles, chronic muscular tension and back pain might be an issue. Athletes in these sports should focus on core strength to assist their balance on the slopes and to support their backs. They should also perform deep and relaxing stretches to offset time spent crouched and controlled.

Strength Focus		
Ab Work (p. 54)		• One breath per movement.
Modified Flow Series (p. 32)	• One breath per movement. • Perform Flow Series instead (p. 32).	
1. Child's Pose (p. 164)		• Sink hips toward heels.
2. Kneeling Plank (p. 40)		• Draw forward with a neutral spine.
3. Kneeling Crocodile (p. 42)		• Lower upper body while lifting abdominals.
4. Cobra (p. 44)		• Lift and open the heart. • Lengthen out of lower back.
5. Child's Pose (p. 164)		• Sink hips toward heels.
Bridge (p. 140)		• Hold for 5-10 breaths.
Bow (p. 138)		• Hold for 5-10 breaths.
Chair (p. 88)		• Hold for 3-5 breaths.

Twisting Chair (p. 150)		• Hold for 3-5 breaths.

Flexibility Focus

Standing Chest Expansion With Forward Fold (p. 116)		• Hold for 3-5 breaths.
Camel (p. 134)		• Hold for 5-10 breaths.
Upside-Down Pigeon (p. 178)		• Hold for 5-10 breaths.
Seated Forward Fold (p. 124)		• Hold for 5-10 breaths.
Quad Stretch (p. 168)		• Hold for 5-10 breaths.
Frog (p. 174)		• Hold for 5-10 breaths.
Butterfly (p. 176)		• Hold for 5-10 breaths.

Additional Practice

- Practice Three-Part breath (p. 22) and other breathing techniques for more efficient, focused, and intense workouts.
- Improve mental game through meditation and visualization.
- Perform any twists (chapter 8).
- Perform any standing balance poses, especially Balancing Half-Moon (p. 94), Tree (p. 96), and Warrior III (p. 90).
- Perform shoulder rolls and stretches.

Weightlifting

Weightlifting, an integral part of most sports and fitness programs, is best complemented by poses that increase flexibility. Incorporating YogaFit poses and sequences into a weightlifting training program promotes healthy joints and strong, flexible muscles and tendons, benefiting athletes and fitness enthusiasts alike.

Between Sets		
Downward-Facing Dog (p. 108)		• Hold for 3-5 breaths.
Bow (p. 138)		• Hold for 5-10 breaths.
Standing Chest Expansion With Forward Fold (p. 116)		• Hold for 3-5 breaths.
Flexibility Focus		
Pyramid (p. 114)		• Hold for 3-5 breaths.
Standing Backbend (p. 130)		• Hold for 3-5 breaths.
Camel (p. 134)		• Hold for 5-10 breaths.
Kneeling Shoulder Stretch (p. 170)		• Hold for 5-10 breaths.

Kickboxing and Boxing

Boxing and kickboxing create tightness in the shoulders and hips and are potentially hard on the knees and back. Because these sports tend to be quite aerobic, athletes should practice deep breathing for maximum efficiency and focus. They can balance the explosive movements of their sports with YogaFit poses that help keep the joints stable and mobile. Flexibility and balance are critical for strength and agility, so boxers and kickboxers should perform deep stretches and standing balance poses regularly.

Strength Focus		
Ab Work (p. 54)		• One breath per movement.
Downward-Facing Dog (p. 108)		• Hold for 3-5 breaths.
Spinal Balance (p. 56)		• Hold for 3-5 breaths.
Flexibility Focus		
Standing Chest Expansion With Forward Fold (p. 116)		• Hold for 3-5 breaths.
Kneeling Shoulder Stretch (p. 170)		• Hold for 5-10 breaths.
Camel (p. 134)		• Hold for 5-10 breaths.
Additional Practice		
• Perform standing balance poses, such as Tree (p. 96), Eagle (p. 98), and Balancing Half-Moon (p. 94).		

Five-Minute Poststretch for Any Sport

Any athlete or "gym-goer" can use this well-rounded stretch following any physical activity. Hold each pose for 5 to 10 breaths (or 5 to 10 breaths on each side, when applicable). See chapter 9 for information on stretching regularly for strength, balance, and flexibility. This workout relieves stress and tension in the lower back, hips, hamstrings, and hip flexors.

Knees to Chest (p. 182)		• Place hands on your hamstrings versus your shins. • Focus on releasing your lower back. • Hold for 5-10 breaths.
Seated Spinal Twist (p. 154)		• Inhale and lengthen; exhale and rotate. • Use your core versus your arm to deepen rotation. • Switch sides. • Hold for 5-10 breaths.
Upside-Down Pigeon (p. 178)		• Flex your feet. • Switch sides. • Hold for 5-10 breaths.
Big Toe Hold (p. 186)		• Keep both hips on the mat, bending knees as necessary. • Switch sides. • Hold each phase for 5 breaths.
Supine Half-Lotus (p. 180)		• Relax completely. • Avoid any position that causes discomfort in the knee. • Switch sides. • Hold for 5-10 breaths.
Bridge or Wheel (p. 140 and 142)	*or*	• Practice Expanding breath. • Slide your shoulders away from your ears. • Follow with Knees to Chest (p. 182). • Hold for 5-10 breaths.

Dead Bug (p. 184)		• Keep your tailbone on the floor. • Stack your ankles over your knees. • Hold for 5-10 breaths.
Butterfly (p. 176)		• Hold Butterfly for 5-10 breaths. • Lie on your back with the soles of your feet together, knees open wide for 5-10 breaths. • Relax completely.
Knees to Chest (p. 182)		• Place your hands on your hamstrings versus your shins. • Focus on releasing your lower back. • Hold for 5-10 breaths.
Fish (p. 194)		• Follows inversions as a counterpose to open throat and chest. • Hold fo 5-10 breaths.
Final Relaxation (p. 196)		• Find a comfortable position that allows you to relax (option: place feet on floor with knees bent). • Let go of distractions. • Let go of controlling your breath. • Hold for as long as time allows.

11

Diet and Nutrition

The foundation of any yoga and fitness practice is a healthy diet that provides nourishment to your body to carry you through your day and through your yoga practice. Without vital nutrients, your body becomes weak and leaves a door open for illness and disease.

The purpose of eating is to create a healthy, strong, and flexible body. Your body supports you in everything you do. When you eat you supply your being with life-force energy called "prana," as you learned in chapter 3 (also called *chi*). Besides nourishing your body, prana also clears your mind and boosts your spirit. You know from experience that when you eat well you feel better on all levels. That's the power of prana. The best nutritional program for those serious about their yoga practice involves simple, fresh, clean, and natural foods.

> Can YogaFit help you lose weight? Absolutely. If you are truly in touch with your body, you will not overindulge or eat unhealthy foods. A YogaFit workout not only makes you sweat, burn calories, and increase your metabolism, it's also widely believed that yoga helps shed pounds through addressing mental and emotional issues. Understanding why you eat is just as important as regulating what you eat and when. The result is a healthier body, mind, and spirit. Take time in your Mountain III poses to practice awareness—not just how you feel, but what you feel and why. Off your mat, use this same awareness to decide what your body really needs and when.

Each day you make important decisions on what to put into your body. Your diet choices either benefit or harm your health. When your daily choices become a lifelong pattern, the benefits or consequences can be significant.

The challenge is to combine foods that are delicious with meals that are nutritionally balanced to sustain your active lifestyle.

EATING A YOGIC DIET

I recently took a trip to India and visited the village of Rishikesh, the birthplace of yoga. While there, I witnessed firsthand the eating habits of yogis. I discovered that alcohol is absent from their diet, and so is meat. Villagers make their meal choices with the health of their bodies *and* their spirits in mind. As discussed in chapter 2, yoga philosophy is based on the Yama *Ahimsa*, the practice of nonviolence and not harming. A vegetarian diet is part of this philosophy.

The traditional yogic diet is vegetarian, promoting nonviolence to ourselves as well as all other living creatures. Yogis believe that our diets should nourish our bodies with foods containing prana, such as pure fruits, grains, and vegetables, while avoiding foods that overstimulate the digestive system. This approach to nutrition is called *sattvic* and involves choosing a diet that's wholesome and pure to promote good health, lightness, and higher consciousness.

The American Dietetic Association (ADA) acknowledges what traditional yogis have known for centuries. Based on medical research, the ADA states that vegetarians have "lower rates of death from ischemic heart disease . . . lower blood cholesterol levels, lower blood pressure, and lower rates of hypertension, type 2 diabetes, and prostate and colon cancer," and that vegetarians are less likely than meat-eaters to be obese. Clearly, excess meat eating can be detrimental to our overall health.

Many Westerners begin yoga with no interest in adopting a vegetarian lifestyle. If that's the case with you, there remain many ways for you to alter your current diet to increase your health and take inches off your waistline. Below are some simple tips from the ADA to get you started on creating a pure and wholesome diet (for more information, see www.eatright.org).

1. Emphasize fruits, vegetables, and whole grains in meals and snacks.
2. Choose proteins such as peanut butter, fish, beans, free-range eggs, and nuts.
3. Choose foods low in saturated fat, trans fats, sodium, and sugar.
4. Vary your veggies. Eat more orange and dark green vegetables such as carrots, sweet potatoes, broccoli, and dark leafy greens. Include pinto beans, kidney beans, split peas, and lentils.
5. Get your calcium-rich foods. Have broccoli, salmon, or the equivalent in yogurt or cheese (a half-ounce of cheese equals one cup of milk). If you choose not to consume milk, choose soy, almond, or rice milk, or eat calcium-fortified foods and beverages.
6. Eat at least half of your daily grains as whole foods, such as whole-grain cereals, rice, and pasta.
7. Go lean with protein. Bake it, broil it, or grill it. Don't fry it.

8. Focus on fresh, frozen, or dried fruits.

9. Avoid canned or packaged foods.

OTHER IDEAS FOR HEALTH

Every day offers you an opportunity to make healthy choices; good health is simply a result of making positive choices on a regular basis. The good news is you get to choose—exercise over being sedentary, water over soda, fresh over fried, and supplements over sugar. Experts say it takes 21 days to form a good habit. Here are some habits worth starting today.

Drink Water

You need to consume fresh water daily, and particularly when engaging in physical activity. As you sweat during your yoga practice, you need to replace your fluids to keep your body in a state of balance and avoid dehydration.

The symptoms of dehydration are easy to detect as long as you stay aware. The first and most obvious sign is thirst, but you should be consuming fluids regularly even before you feel thirsty. Your body doesn't send the thirst signal until after you've entered the first stage of dehydration. So if you're feeling thirsty, grab your water bottle. If you ignore your thirst, you might progress into the later stages of dehydration (weakness, exhaustion, and delirium).

How much water to drink varies from person to person. The recommended fluid intake for a person expending 2,000 calories a day is 7 to 11 cups. Most of your fluid should be water, however your total intake can include other beverages without caffeine, alcohol, or excess sugar, such as decaffeinated tea and fruit juice. But the ideal amount varies depending on diet, amount of physical activity, environmental temperature, and other factors. Your doctor can best advise you how much to drink and what beverages are most appropriate for you.

The following is a list of fluid-rich foods that contain over 80 percent water. As part of your daily nutritional intake, these foods will help you stay hydrated.

- Berries
- Milk
- Watermelon
- Lettuce
- Cabbage
- Celery
- Spinach
- Broccoli
- Fruit juices (drink in moderation because of the sugars)

- Yogurt
- Apples
- Grapes
- Oranges

Read Labels

In general, most of us need to be more conscious when we shop for our foods. For one thing, we should all understand the catch phrases and labels on foods so that we can make educated choices while shopping. Again, too, we would like to reiterate that you should avoid packaged or canned foods whenever possible. Listed here are the most common phrases you'll see stamped on some of your favorite food items—and what they really mean.

- *Light*—one-third fewer calories or half the amount of fat than the usual food.
- *Low calorie*—fewer than 40 calories per serving.
- *Calorie free*—fewer than 5 calories per serving.
- *Fat free*—less than one-fourth gram of fat per serving.
- *Sugar free*—less than one-fourth gram of sugar per serving.
- *Reduced*—25 percent less of the specified nutrient than the usual product.
- *Good source of*—provides at least 10 percent of the daily value of a particular vitamin or nutrient per serving.
- *High in*—provides more than 20 percent of the daily value of a specified nutrient per serving.
- *Low sodium*—less than 140 milligrams of sodium per serving.
- *Low cholesterol*—less than 20 milligrams of cholesterol and 2 grams or less of saturated fat per serving.
- *Organic*—grown free from antibiotics or pesticides.

Get Plenty of Vitamins and Minerals

Poor nutrition is a common cause of a weakened immune response, and a weakened immune system leaves the body vulnerable to virtually every type of illness and disease, especially during seasonal shifts when coughs and colds are rampant. Fatigue, lethargy, repeated infections, slow wound healing, allergies, thrush, colds, and flu are all signs that the body's immune system is functioning below par. Getting enough rest; eating healthy foods; avoiding excess alcohol, caffeine, and stimulants; exercising; and practicing meditation and introspection are crucial in helping you maintain your optimal health.

Eating lots of fruits and vegetables should pay off for your immune system. Fruits and vegetables contain hundreds of phytochemicals that provide many preventative health benefits. They are also excellent sources of carotenoids, which boost the activity of white blood cells called lymphocytes. Beta-carotene (from carrots and elsewhere) can also be converted to vitamin A in your body, an important nutrient for the immune system. Organic fruits and vegetables are always a wise choice.

Natural sources of immune-boosting antioxidants include kiwi fruit, which contains more vitamin C than oranges; Chinese cabbage, an excellent source of vitamin A; and avocado, known as nature's own super food because it provides the optimal ratio of fat, carbohydrate, protein, and vitamin E. Foods rich in vitamin B6, which boosts the production of antibodies to fight infection, are also good choices. These include bananas, carrots, lentils, tuna, salmon, whole-grain flour, and sunflower seeds. Many people also need to increase their intake of dietary zinc by eating more seafood, eggs, turkey, pumpkin seeds, and crabmeat.

Here are some practical tips for boosting your immune system:

- *Take echinacea when your immune system is weak.* You might have heard of this best-selling herbal remedy, which is prescribed in Germany by doctors and pharmacists to help fight colds and flu. This herb is effective as long as you don't overuse it; take it during times of immune stress, such as when traveling, during the winter, or when you're working out a lot.

- *Consume plenty of vitamin C.* Vitamin C, a nutrient commonly associated with preventing colds, has a widespread reputation as an immunity booster. Most people reach for vitamin C tablets at the first sign of a cold. Many of the symptoms of a cold, however, have nothing to do with the cold virus itself but are caused by the body's own immune response to the alien invader. It's this secondary problem that vitamin C helps to counter. Don't underestimate the importance of consuming good food sources of vitamin C. Many endurance athletes consume over three servings of fresh fruit and up to two cups of cooked vegetables daily for ample amounts of dietary vitamin C. Most research measuring the effects of high doses of vitamin C through supplementation have not shown additional protection to the immune system, though many athletes swear by their vitamin C supplements. What we do know is that a daily dose of 250 milligrams is adequate to saturate your body stores with vitamin C. Excellent sources of vitamin C include sweet peppers, citrus fruits and juices, strawberries, cantaloupe, kiwi fruit, and broccoli.

- *Eat foods with natural sources of vitamin E.* Vitamin E is an antioxidant and nutrient that slows down the process of aging and strengthens body cells that fight infection. People who eat foods rich in vitamin E have an added weapon against bacteria and viruses. Vitamin E also helps in the fight against heart disease and cancer. Good food sources of vitamin E are whole-grain foods and vegetable oils. If you're not getting enough of this vitamin in your meals, supplements can help you reach the daily requirement. Check with your doctor about dosage.

- *Consume folate.* Found in orange juice, spinach, beans, and fortified grain products, folate might help lower inflammation. A lack of folate in adults has been associated with a higher risk for certain types of cancers. Adequate folate intake is also recommended for all women of childbearing age, whether they're planning to become pregnant or not. Folate is essential in preventing defects to a baby's spine during the first days and weeks of pregnancy.

- *Choose foods containing flavonoids.* Found in plant foods such as citrus fruits, berries, and some vegetables, flavonoids function as antioxidants. Scientists believe flavonoids might help reduce the risk of cancer, heart disease, and other serious health problems.

- *Consume zinc, iron, and vitamins B6 and B12.* These are nutrients essential for a strong immune system. A well-balanced diet and a daily multivitamin and mineral supplement that provides 100 percent of the daily values of these nutrients should ensure adequate intake. Don't overdo it with these nutrients. Megadosing with vitamins and minerals can compromise the immune system (especially if you take too much iron), impair immune function, and increase susceptibility to infection. Although iron is an essential mineral, iron supplements should be taken as required with regular monitoring. Excess iron can increase inflammation in the body. Research on zinc supplementation and the common cold is split down the middle in regards to effectiveness. Limited evidence suggests that zinc supplements can reduce the severity or duration of a cold, but the zinc must be taken within 24 hours of the onset of symptoms to provide any benefit.

- *Eat your omega 3s.* Polyunsaturated oils that provide omega-6 and omega-3 fatty acids are good for the immune system. Most North Americans consume enough of the omega-6 fats (if not an excess) but need to increase their intake of omega-3s. Walnuts, fatty fish (salmon, sardines) and flax, soy, and canola oils are good sources of this healthy fat.

A proper balance of the right kind of fat in your diet can boost your immune system. A very high-fat diet can compromise immune function, but a very low-fat diet doesn't provide adequate amounts of essential fatty acids.

Another thing to consider, especially if you're considering changing your diet to lose weight: Rapid weight loss of greater than two pounds per week (an amount often recommended by diet programs) can have negative effects on your immune system. If you're an athlete, you especially want to take care in any weight-reduction plan. Consuming adequate calories is beneficial for your recovery and energy levels. Diets too low in energy might cause inadequate intake of immune-boosting vitamins and minerals. Poorly planned and low-calorie diets can also be low in protein, and a low-protein diet can compromise your immune system.

NUTRITIONAL STRATEGIES FOR TRAINING AND WORKING OUT

Periods of heavy physical activity are associated with a depressed immune function, and compromised immune function is aggravated by inadequate nutrition. Your body's susceptibility to a respiratory infection can be elevated for 24 hours after a tough workout, whereas a demanding race might impair your immune function for one to two weeks. Further, if you're an endurance athlete, combining training with a heavy workload can overtax your resources, stress your body, and compromise your ability to fight infection.

Because increased oxygen use during exercise can increase the production of free radicals (unstable molecules that can cause tissue damage at the cellular level), increased food intake and supplementation with antioxidants might enhance immune-system performance. Consume a healthy diet and supplement wisely, though. When your immune system is compromised from training, this effect is related to elevated concentrations of stress hormones. Consuming carbohydrates before, during, and after physical activity—a familiar practice for endurance athletes—appears to diminish some of the immunosuppressive effects of intense training. Carbohydrate intake before, during, and after activity results in lower cortisol levels, fewer changes in blood immune cell counts, lower oxidative activity, and a diminished inflammatory response.

So practicing yoga with optimal stores of carbohydrate not only provides fuel for your workout but also supports a strong immune system. On the other hand, training in a carbohydrate-depleted state can cause greater increases in the stress hormones that increase during exercise.

The nutritional strategies presented here, combined with a regular yoga practice, adequate rest, and time out for meditation and relaxation, can have a dramatic impact on your health and well-being. Healthy habits regarding nutrition might also move you to make more dramatic changes to your diet and lifestyle, such as becoming a vegetarian. However, if you feel overwhelmed at the thought of making major changes overnight, keep in mind that yoga is meant to be a process. Every change, no matter how small, can make a difference. Take one step at a time, listen to your body, and the rewards you receive will be enough to inspire you to keep moving forward on your journey to a stronger and healthier mind, body, and spirit.

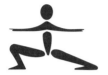

12

Meditation

Much of our daily life is spent in our heads, focused on what we're thinking rather than on what we're feeling. With all the demands of work and home we're often required to stay one mental step ahead just to get through the day. The problem is, when we navigate through life led by our thoughts alone, we miss out on a world of information available to us through our bodies and spirits.

The ancient practice of meditation is as integral to yoga as the poses are, and they have the same intention: not to tune out, but to tune in to a frequency long forgotten, or perhaps undiscovered. To meditate is to become acutely aware of what's going on within you; it's about learning to tame your mind so that you can focus all your energy and awareness on the task at hand. The practice of meditation helps you stay centered regardless of your circumstances. It doesn't teach you to avoid pain or discomfort but to experience and accept it so you can move through any situation with profound clarity and a sense of inner peace and calm. Meditation is a wonderful way to tap into your internal knowingness and stay in touch with your eternal essence.

Meditation at first can be awkward and unfamiliar. It might be eye-opening to discover you are controlled by incessant thoughts, and it might be frustrating to realize that many of them are unnecessary and perhaps even based in misperception or falsehood. Sitting in silence, you might realize how many common distractions compete for your attention, including doubt, sleepiness, and restlessness. Rather than using up even more energy in fighting these hindrances, you eventually realize it's far easier to acknowledge them and release them. Distractions will never let up, but you can teach yourself to let them go. In fact, an awareness of your thought life and distractions is the first step toward developing a successful meditation practice that will improve your physical and mental well-being.

When you refine your ability to slip into a state of awareness and being, you can bring this focus into other areas of your life. No matter what's happening in your immediate environment, you can step back and respond rather than react. Whether it's an athletic competition, work, a difficult conversation, or a game you're playing, you will enjoy what you're doing much more, and perhaps even do it much better.

So give yourself permission to be a beginner, and know that with practice your ability to concentrate will improve. Eventually, you'll find that during meditation you might slip between thoughts, or you might discover yourself unaware of any thoughts at all. In this place, you might not only lose track of what you hear around you but discover you've lost all sense of time. With practice, you'll find that you can meditate in a noisy airport or on a busy street corner without becoming distracted.

> You are not seeking to find anything through the practice of meditation. Rather, it is through meditation that you are found. It's a mistake to think that through meditation you are trying to become somebody else. The true intent of yoga and meditation is to become the best possible version of yourself.

BENEFITS OF MEDITATION

Because practicing meditation helps you to slow your breath, quiet your mind, and find peace, it can be beneficial physically, mentally, and emotionally. Meditation is now commonly used to treat mental health disorders, addiction, and everyday stress, as well as to heal physical ailments and promote better sleep.

Physical Benefits

- Stimulates your parasympathetic nervous system, or the branch of your peripheral nervous system that helps your body return to a calm, relaxed state after the threat of danger, or even daily stress, has passed. When this branch is activated, your body can naturally rejuvenate, repair, and rebuild itself.
- Clears your mind for better quality sleep.
- Improves athletic performance by refining your ability to focus on a goal or situation (another term for meditation used in this way is visualization).
- Slows your respiration for longer, deeper breaths.
- Boosts your immune system by slowing the production of the stress hormone cortisol.

Mental and Emotional Benefits

- Reduces anxiety and depression by enabling your body to balance its own neurochemical system.
- Allows you to make better decisions and improve critical thinking.
- Breaks unhealthy habits by helping you detach emotions associated with an action from the action itself.
- Improves communication with yourself. When you better understand your thought processes, you have more control over what you think.
- Helps you stay in the present moment. When you let go of the past and the future, you live 100 percent in the now, which affects all aspects of your life and relationships.

ACTIVE MEDITATION TECHNIQUES

There are many different meditation traditions and techniques. Westerners, accustomed to fast-paced living and constant information exchange, often benefit more from active meditation techniques. Active meditation involves focusing your thoughts and awareness on a particular thought, idea, visualization, or concept. Choosing to focus on something positive can help you rid your mind of negative thoughts and emotions and other clutter. Whatever your meditation practice looks like, be sure to embrace the essence of YogaFit: Let go of all judgment of your experience.

Here are some steps to help you establish a personal active meditation practice:

1. Commit to meditating at least 10 minutes every day (more, if possible). Set an alarm so you don't have to keep an eye on the clock. To help make your meditation practice a habit, practice at the same time each day, or establish a routine, such as meditating immediately after your YogaFit session. Finally, if you have room, establish a special place to sit and meditate at home. Place a chair in a corner near a favorite window, or surround a cushion with your favorite candles—try to create your own sacred space. Knowing you have somewhere you love to go will help you get there.

2. Whether you're in a chair, on a cushion, or on the floor, sit *comfortably* with your spine straight. If you're not comfortable, you'll be distracted. If you're practicing before or after your YogaFit workout, roll up your mat and sit on it; elevating your hips eases tension in your hips and hamstrings and improves circulation to your legs.

3. Use the Relaxation breath technique (p. 23). Sitting upright with a neutral spine, relax your abdomen and breathe quietly without forcing your exhalations. Take the same amount of time for your inhale and your exhale, consciously beginning your inhale just as your exhale ends. Your abdominal

muscles must not be constrained by tension or clothing; you must be completely free to move.

4. Select one of the following techniques. If the technique you choose doesn't work, let it go and try another.

- Choose a *mantra* (word or phrase), thought, or feeling on which to meditate. Repeat your mantra over and over in rhythm with your breath. If your first choice leads to negative thoughts or feelings, let it go and choose something else. For example, a common mantra is "om" (pronounced Aaaaaah Ooooo Mmmmmm), which represents the root of all sounds that are ever-present as vibrations in your body.

- Visualize an object or place in which you find peace, such as a lotus blossom or a quiet beach.

- If preparing for a performance or competition, visualize yourself succeeding; use all your senses as you mentally act out the scenario.

- Use a guided meditation. Many such meditations are available on CD. Relax and fully listen to each word.

- Use an affirmation card with a phrase that inspires or strengthens you. Many books and box sets with positive affirmations are available. Or you can make your own.

- Focus on a small, meaningful object held in your hand or placed in front you.

5. After meditating, reflect on the experience in a journal. For example, write down any techniques you tried and what you experienced practicing them. What were your thoughts and feelings before, during, and after meditating? Also note if you made any headway toward working out questions or situations you've struggled to resolve. Finally, keep track of the benefits you notice from incorporating meditation into your yoga practice. These will become incentives to continue.

RECOGNIZING YOUR SUCCESS

How do you know if you're meditating successfully? People describe their meditative states in a wide variety of ways. Some see a single source of light, some see themselves from a distance, and others see images or even sense colors. Some people see or feel nothing they can express in words. Some experience a wonderful state of beingness, an inner glow of warmth and peace. All these experiences indicate a successful meditation session. Just as there's no best version of a yoga pose, there's no one best way to meditate.

As you explore the meditation techniques described in this chapter, remember that every day is different and every session is different; you're constantly faced with new struggles and challenges. Yet your inner truths remain the same; you need only to look within. Whatever your meditation looks or feels like, remember to embrace the essence of YogaFit and let go of all expectations.

APPENDIX A

THE CHAKRAS

The word "chakra" is Sanskrit for wheel or disk. There are seven basic chakra energy centers, or nerve bundles, along the spinal column, as shown in figure A1. Each of these centers correlates to major nerve ganglia branching forth from the spinal column and has a corresponding relationship to one of the glands of the body's endocrine system. Each chakra stimulates different organs and systems in the body. The first six chakras begin at the coccyx and continue up to the cervical vertebrae, while the seventh chakra is associated with the cerebral cortex of the brain.

Hatha yoga exercises, like the ones we use in YogaFit, activate these energy centers by their very nature to enhance overall balance and performance. Moving the spine keeps the nerve impulses flowing. The following warm-up and workout formats are designed to target the seven different chakras in your

Spinal Column/Nerves	Seven Chakras/Nerve Bundles	YogaFit Energy Centers
	Chakra Seven – Cerebral Cortex	Crown Center
	Chakra Six – Carotid Plexus	Brow Center
	Chakra Five – Pharyngeal Plexus	Throat Center
	Chakra Four – Pulmonary and Cardiac Plexus	Heart Center
	Chakra Three – Solar Plexus	Solar Plexus Center
	Chakra Two – Sacral Plexus	Navel Center
	Chakra One – Coccygeal Plexus	Root Center

body to help them function correctly and prevent nerve bundles from getting blocked. Traditionally, the chakras are also associated with various issues and concepts associated with our mental, emotional, and spiritual life. The chart below serves as a brief and general introduction to these associations; it also indicates each chakra's corresponding color. To learn more about the chakras and how they relate to you, order YogaFit's *Chakra Balancing Kit* listed in the Recommended Reading section of appendix B.

The YogaFit Chakra Energy Warm-Up

First chakra	Moonflowers (p. 68)
Second chakra	Sunflowers (p. 70)
Third chakra	Chair Flow (described in Standard Standing Warm-Up and Standard Lying Down Warm-Up on pp. 204-207)
Fourth chakra	Cat and Cow (described in Standard Standing Warm-Up and Standard Lying Down Warm-Up on pp. 204-207)
Fifth chakra	Plank Push-Up Series (described in the Flex and Flow workout on p. 212)
Sixth chakra	Modified Flow Series (p. 32)
Seventh chakra	Spinal Balance (described in Standard Standing Warm-Up and Standard Lying Down Warm-Up on pp. 204-207)

Chakra Energy Workout

Chakra	Physical focus	Mental/emotional/ spiritual focus	Color visualization
Chakra 1: *Root*	Mountain Pose (p. 66) and breathing (see chapter 3)	Grounding	Red
Chakra 2: *Navel*	Flow sequences	Creativity/flow/sensuality	Orange
Chakra 3: *Solar plexus*	Mountain II poses, such as Warrior I (p. 76), Warrior II (p. 78), Warrior III (p. 90), and Reverse Warrior (p. 80)	Discipline, willpower, personal power	Yellow
Chakra 4: *Heart*	Expansion poses, such as Camel (p. 134), Standing Backbend (p. 130), and Chest Expansion With Forward Fold (p. 116)	Love, self-acceptance, agape	Green
Chakra 5: *Throat*	Chanting or mantras (see chapter 12)	Communication	Blue
Chakra 6: *Third eye*	Creative visualization (see chapter 12)	Insight/vision	Purple
Chakra 7: *Crown*	Meditation (see chapter 12)	Unification with higher self and universe	White

APPENDIX B

RECOMMENDED READING & SHOPPING

Beth has selected a variety of books and other tools to broaden your understanding of yoga and other related mind–body topics. To order the books listed here or for more titles, visit our Web site at www.yogafit.com.

- *Therapeutic Yoga for the Shoulders and Hips,* Susi Hately Aldous
- *Yoga as Medicine: The Yogic Prescription for Health and Healing,* Timothy McCall
- *Anatomy and Asana,* Susi Hately Aldous
- *Chakra Meditation,* Swami Saradananda
- *Chakra Balancing,* Kit Anondea Judith
- *Creative Visualization* (book and workbook), Shakti Gawain
- *Eating Mindfully,* Susan Albers
- *Natural Prozac,* Joel Robertson
- *Pathways to Joy,* edited by Dave Deluca
- *The Power of Now* (book and inspiration deck), Eckhart Tolle
- *The Key Muscles of Hatha Yoga,* Ray Long
- *The Language of Yoga,* Nicolai Bachman
- *The Living Gita,* Sri Swami Satchidananda
- *The Mandala of Being,* Richard Moss
- *The Yoga Sutras of Patanjali,* Sri Swami Satchidananda
- *Your Body Speaks Your Mind,* Deb Shapiro
- *Growing the Positive Mind,* William K. Larkin

YogaFit continues to produce DVDs for every level, from *YogaFit Basics* to *Active Advanced,* as well as DVDs for specialty populations, including *YogaFit Plus* for larger bodies, *YogaFit Seniors, YogaFit Kids,* and *YogaFit Prenatal/Postpartum.* To order or to get more information on which formats are most appropriate for you, visit our Web site at www.yogafit.com.

YogaFit also provides CDs to enhance your YogaFit experience. Our Active, Slow Flow, and Zen Series CDs are compiled to correspond with the Three Mountain model of warm-up, work, and cool-down. Our collection includes a variety of artists and styles so you can find the perfect music for your practice or class. To order, listen to CDs, or find out more about which formats are most appropriate for you, visit our Web site at www.yogafit.com.

Since its inception, YogaFit has offered high-quality, high-performance clothing and accessories at competitive prices. Bulk pricing is available on all YogaFit products. Just order a minimum of 12 pieces (per style) or items and receive incredible savings. To order or view photographs of our clothing line, as well as our mats, blocks, straps, and more, visit www.yogafit.com.

APPENDIX C

YOGAFIT TEACHER TRAINING & PARTNERING PROGRAM

YogaFit is committed to providing you with the best educational and business opportunities to further your knowledge and teaching opportunities within the YogaFitness Industry. In what follows you'll find information about YogaFit's Teacher Training Program and YogaFit's Partnering Program.

YogaFit's Teacher Training Program

YogaFit, the company, and its teacher training program have expanded considerably over the years and now feature internationally renowned certification programs for fitness professionals. YogaFit has trained over 100,000 fitness professionals and yoga instructors at facilities in the United States and internationally, and has been integral in the practice of yoga becoming a primary part of health club, gym, and spa programs throughout the world.

YogaFit offers over 25 different educational trainings and a broad spectrum of specialty programs so you can choose how deep you want to delve. You are welcome to explore the many diverse aspects of the discipline of yoga from an open, objective perspective that focuses on holistic (mind–body) health benefits through YogaFit. Yogafit runs ten Mind/Body/Fitness Conferences (MBFs) per year nationwide. These conferences offer all levels of training plus specialty programming. A fun and interactive way to learn, MBFs offer speakers, raffles, gift bags, and group bonding. YogaFit's Corporate Headquarters is located in Torrance, California. There are YogaFit Studio Partners across the world. YogaFit has trained instructors in every continent and continues to expand the horizons of fitness professionals and other individuals around the globe.

Taught by YogaFit-trained instructors with in-depth experience and skills in both yoga and fitness, the YogaFit method is a nationally recognized continuing education credit provider for the American Council on Exercise (ACE) and has been a member of IHRSA since 1997. YogaFit is also the only yoga instruction certified by Town Sports International (TSI) and New York, Washington, Boston, and Philadelphia Fitness Clubs. Team YogaFit currently has 50 trainers internationally.

The YogaFit Teacher Trainings are typically one to four days of high-quality, hands-on instruction and team teaching; the program provides enough support material to allow you to start your first class right away. Training classes are held in many locations throughout the United States and other countries. For more details, visit www.yogafit.com.

Community Service Mission and Conscious Business Paradigm

YogaFit is dedicated to community service via community outreach programs from their corporate headquarters and partner studios. We believe that if everyone in the world gave one hour per week of community service work, the world would be a better place. This is why we require every YogaFit Level One trainee to perform eight hours of practice teaching in a community service setting before receiving a Certificate of Completion. Our trainees have brought the practice and benefits of yoga to seniors in long-term care homes, stressed-out corporate executives, cancer patients and survivors, disabled persons, incarcerated persons, terminally ill persons, children, mentally challenged individuals, and military servants, just to name a few.

The Community Service Program gives our trainees the opportunity to practice their new teaching skills in a less stressful environment with an appreciative audience. As the thousands of letters we receive in our corporate office attest to, volunteering time and energy has proven to be the most rewarding experience for many of our trainees. YogaFit is dedicated to this work because it promotes the essence of giving and sharing freely.

YogaFit is a green company and encourages green business practices. YogaFit also encourages and supports the philosophy of Conscious Business. In this millennium we believe the companies that are socially responsible will prosper from good will and good karma. Together we are changing the paradigm of what it means to do good business . . . really *good* business.

YogaFit's Partners and Partner Program

Are you YogaFit-trained and want to call your classes YogaFit? Then the YogaFit Partner Program is for you. This program allows either a club or studio owner employing YogaFit-trained instructors, or individual YogaFit-trained instructors themselves, to partner with YogaFit and use the powerful YogaFit brand name in marketing your services (only applies to accounts within the United States). Just send us your name, facility, phone, fax number, and e-mail, and we'll get back to you with details. We look forward to working with you, and having you join the YogaFit team of Partners. Visit our Web site at www.yogafit.com for more details.

YogaFit Club Series (YCS)

The YogaFit Club Series offers prechoreographed workouts for health clubs and spas to take the guesswork and liability out of their yoga classes. YCS offers DVDs, CDs, and workout formats to participating clubs and instructors.

Yoga Alliance

Through YogaFit's comprehensive 200- and 500-hour teacher training programs, you can become a registered yoga teacher (RYT) with the Yoga Alliance, a nonprofit organization that supports yoga teachers and upholds the diversity and integrity of yoga. This certification gives you the professional credibility and experience now sought by health clubs and studios. Please visit our Web site at www.yogafit.com to view the educational requirements to obtain your Yoga Alliance RYT certificate through YogaFit.

The American Council on Exercise (ACE)

YogaFit has chosen the American Council on Exercise (ACE) as its premier provider of fitness certifications. ACE is the only certifying body to offer four fitness certifications accredited by the National Commission for Certifying Agencies (NCCA): (1) group exercise instructor; (2) personal trainer; (3) lifestyle weight management; and (4) clinical exercise specialist.

POSE INDEX

ABOUT
THE AUTHOR

Beth Shaw, E-RYT, BS, CMT, is the president and founder of YogaFit Training Systems Inc. The leader in mind–body education, YogaFit has trained more than 75,000 fitness instructors on six continents. Shaw is an internationally known fitness expert and the author of *Beth Shaw's Yogafit* (Human Kinetics, 2001) and the publisher of *Angles* magazine, which is distributed to yoga fitness enthusiasts and instructors. Shaw and her company have been showcased in numerous fitness magazines as well as *Time*, *More*, *Entrepreneur*, *Yoga Journal*, and *USA Today*. She has also been featured on CNBC, CNN, NBC, CBS, E Style Channel, Showtime, and *Donny Deutsch's Big Idea*.

Ms. Shaw is an innovative educator, entrepreneur, and visionary responsible for YogaFit as well as YogaButt, YogaStrength, YogaCore, Yoga Lean, and count-

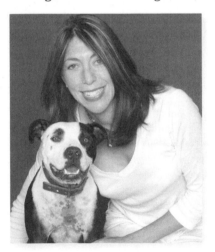

less other yoga fitness combinations. She has more than 30 DVDs and CDs on the market and is widely recognized as the premier yoga fitness trainer in the fitness industry.

Ms. Shaw is also known for her community service initiatives. As an animal rights activist, Shaw serves on the National Council for the Humane Society of the United States and is the chairperson for Karma Rescue, a Los Angeles-based dog rescue that supports many animal rescue groups. Her nonprofit organization, Visionary Women in Fitness, awards scholarships and grants to women in need. She lives in Redondo Beach, California.